Springer Series on the Teaching of Nursing

Diane O. McGivern, RN, PhD, FAAN, Series Editor
New York University Division of Nursing

Advisory Board: Ellen Baer, PhD, RN, FAAN; Carla Mariano, EdD, RN;
Janet A. Rodgers, PhD, RN, FAAN; Alice Adam Young, PhD, RN

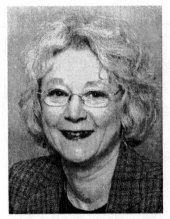

Lois K. Evans is Viola MacInnes/Independence Professor at the University of Pennsylvania School of Nursing where she facilitated the development of the School's network of community based nursing practices—the Penn Nursing Network and provided leadership for the School's evolving agenda to integrate its missions for research, education and clinical care. She also co-directed the Penn-Macy Initiative to Advance Academic Nursing Practice. In addition to models of health care, Dr. Evans research interests focus on indvidualized care for frail elders, including restraint reduction and behavior in dementia; culture, environments, and quality of care and quality of life in nursing homes, and recognition and management of depression in older adults. She has received numerous awards for her research on individualized care and restraint use with frail elders and is an elected Fellow in the American Academy of Nursing and the Gerontological Society of America. Dr. Evans is Co-Director of the School's Center for Gerontologic Nursing Science and the John A. Hartford Center of Geriatric Nursing Excellence, Chairs the Family and Community Health Division, Co-Directs the Delaware Valley Geriatric Education Center and teaches in the geropsychiatric graduate nursing program.

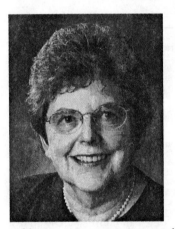

Norma M. Lang is Lillian Brunner Professor of Medical Surgical Nursing at the University of Pennsylvania School of Nursing. She is a Senior Research Fellow in the Annenberg Public Policy Center and a Senior Fellow in the Leonard Davis Institute for Health Economics. She directs the Office of International Programs and the WHO/PAHO Collaborating Center for Nursing and Midwifery Leadership. She is the Dean Emeritus of Nursing (1992-2000) and former Dean and Professor at the University of Wisconsin-Milwaukee School of Nursing (1980-1992). Dr. Lang's research interests include quality assurance, nursing standards and outcome measures, peer review, the Nursing Minimum Data Set and the development of the International Classification for Nursing Practice. She has authored numerous publications. Her pioneering work in identifying standards and measures to evaluate the quality of nursing care has served as a basis for nursing policy throughout the world. The seminal model for measuring and evaluating the quality of nursing care that bears her name has been adopted in several countries. Her teaching expertise is in executive management, leadership, informatics, and classification for nursing practice. She has been an advisor and faculty member for the Wharton Johnson & Johnson (J & J) Program in Management for Nurse Executives and co-directed the Penn Macy Institute to Advance Academic Nursing Practice. Dr. Lang is a fellow of the Institute of Medicine, the American Academy of Nursing, the College of Physicians of Philadelphia and an honorary Fellow of the Royal College of Nursing in London. She was awarded honorary membership in the American Association of Colleges of Nurses. She is the 2001 recipient of the Joint Commission on the Accreditation of Health Care Organizations Ernest A. Codman Award. In 2002 she received the Jessie S. Scott Award from the American Nurses Association.

ACADEMIC NURSING PRACTICE

Lois K. Evans, DNSc, FAAN, RN
Norma M. Lang, PhD, FAAN, FRCN, RN
Editors

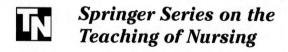

Springer Series on the Teaching of Nursing

3-05

Springer Publishing Company, Inc.
536 Broadway
New York, NY 10012-3955

Acquisitions Editor: Ruth Chasek
Production Editor: Janice Stangel
Cover design by Joanne Honigman

04 05 06 07 08 / 5 4 3 2 1

Library of Congress Cataloging-in-Publication Data

Academic nursing practice : helping to shape the future of healthcare / Lois K. Evans, Norma M. Lang, editors.
    p. ; cm.
  Includes bibliographical references and index.
  ISBN 0-8261-2044-X
  1. Nursing—Study and teaching—United States.
  2. Nursing—United States—Quality control. I. Evans, Lois K.
II. Lang, Norma M.
    [DNLM: 1. Education, Nursing—methods. 2. Clinical Competence.
3. Teaching—methods. WY 18 A168 2004]
RT79.A143 2004
610.73'071'1—dc22   2003067309

Printed in the United States of America by Integrated Book Technology.

To all deans, faculty, staff, students, and supporters who are success-fully pioneering in the integration of nursing education, research and practice to improve health care for people in the 21st century.

And to our spouses William Middleton and Glenn Lang whose pa-tience, support, and cheerleading have helped sustain us throughout the experiences detailed in this book, and in finally putting it on paper for all to share.

Contents

List of Tables and Figures

TABLES

FIGURES

Contributors

Betty S. Adler, Esquire
Senior Counsel
Office of the General Counsel
University of Pennsylvania
Philadelphia, Pennsylvania

Linda H. Aiken, PhD, FAAN,
  FRCN, RN
Claire M. Fagin Leadership
  Professor in Nursing
Professor of Sociology
Director
Center for Health Outcomes and
  Policy Research
School of Nursing
University of Pennsylvania
Philadelphia, Pennsylvania

Marina C. Barnett, DSW
Assistant Professor
School of Social Administration
Department of Social Work
Temple University
Philadelphia, Pennsylvania

Jane H. Barnsteiner, PhD, FAAN,
  RN
Professor of Pediatric Nursing
Division Chair Family and
  Community Health
School of Nursing
University of Pennsylvania
Philadelphia, Pennsylvania

Patricia Chiverton, EdD, RN,
  FNAP
Dean and Professor of Nursing
Vice President
Strong Health
School of Nursing
University of Rochester
Rochester, New York

Colleen Conway-Welch, PhD,
  CNM, FAAN
Professor and Dean
Vanderbilt University School of
  Nursing
Nashville, Tennessee

Margaret M. Cotroneo, PhD, RN,
  CS
Associate Professor of Psychiatric
  Mental Health Nursing
School of Nursing
University of Pennsylvania
Philadelphia, Pennsylvania
Former Faculty Director
The Health Annex at the Francis J.
  Myers Recreation Center
Philadelphia, Pennsylvania

Jeffrey Gilbert, BS, CPIHMS
Senior IT Consultant and Partner
Zinganee Associates, LLC
Former Senior IT Project Manager
Penn Nursing Network (PNN)
Philadelphia, Pennsylvania

Susan Greenbaum, BA
Senior Producer
Radio Times
WHYY-FM Public Radio
Philadelphia, Pennsylvania
Former Director of Public
    Relations
School of Nursing
University of Pennsylvania
Philadelphia, Pennsylvania

Margaret Grey, DrPH, CPNP,
    CDE, FAAN
Independence Foundation
    Professor of Nursing
Associate Dean for Research
    Affairs
School of Nursing
Yale University
New Haven, Connecticut

Tine Hansen-Turton, MPA
Executive Director
National Nursing Centers
    Consortium
Philadelphia, Pennsylvania

Melinda Jenkins, PhD, AP, RN
Assistant Professor of Clinical
    Nursing
Family Nurse Practitioner
School of Nursing
Columbia University
Former Assistant Professor of
    Primary Care
School of Nursing
University of Pennsylvania
Philadelphia, Pennsylvania

Catherine R. Judge, BA
Director of Financial Development
Red Cross of Southeastern
    Pennsylvania
Former Assistant Dean for
    Development and Alumni
    Relations
School of Nursing
University of Pennsylvania
Philadelphia, Pennsylvania

Lenore H. Kurlowicz, PhD, RN,
    CS
Assistant Professor of
    Geropsychiatric Nursing
School of Nursing
University of Pennsylvania
Philadelphia, Pennsylvania

Jeffrey S. Levitt, MBA
Chairman and CEO
Precyse Solutions, LLC
Former Member, Board of
    Overseers
School of Nursing
University of Pennsylvania
Philadelphia, Pennsylvania

Terri H. Lipman, PhD, CRNP,
    FAAN
Associate Professor of Nursing of
    Children
School of Nursing
University of Pennsylvania
Philadelphia, Pennsylvania
Pediatric Nurse Practitioner
Endocrinology at Children's
    Hospital of Philadelphia
Philadelphia, Pennsylvania

Joan E. Lynaugh, PhD, RN, FAAN
Professor Emeritus and Associate
    Director of the Center for the
    Study of the History of Nursing
School of Nursing
University of Pennsylvania
Philadelphia, Pennsylvania

Karen Dorman Marek, PhD, MBA, RN, FAAN
Director
University Nurses Senior Care
Sinclair School of Nursing
University of Missouri-Columbia
Former Assistant Professor
School of Nursing
University of Pennsylvania
Philadelphia, Pennsylvania

Danielle C. Martin, DHS
Executive Director
Southwest Community Services, Inc.
Philadelphia, Pennsylvania

Maureen P. McCausland, DNSc, RN, FAAN
Professor of Nursing
    Administration
School of Nursing
University of Pennsylvania
Philadelphia, Pennsylvania
Former Associate Dean for
    Nursing Practice and Former
    Chief Nursing Executive
University of Pennsylvania Health
    System
Philadelphia, Pennsylvania

Anne M. McGinley, PhD, RN
Director
Undergraduate Program
Thomas Jefferson Department of
    Nursing
College of Health
Philadelphia, Pennsylvania
Former Assistant Professor and
    PNNCIS Project Director
School of Nursing
University of Pennsylvania
Philadelphia, Pennsylvania

Barbara Medoff-Cooper, PhD, CRNP, FAAN, RN
Helen M. Shearer Term Professor
    in Nutrition
Director of the Center for Nursing
    Research
School of Nursing
University of Pennsylvania
Philadelphia, Pennsylvania

Kathryn M. Mershon, MSN, CNAA, RN, FAAN
The Mershon Company
Louisville, Kentucky
Former APM Consultant

Bert Orlov, MBA
President
FilmSnacks
Former APM Consultant
New York, New York

Rebecca A. Snyder Phillips, MSN
Director
PNN Consulting/GNCS
Penn Nursing Network
School of Nursing
University of Pennsylvania
Philadelphia, Pennsylvania

Bonita Ann Pilon, DSN, CNAA, FAAN
Professor
Senior Associate Dean
Practice Management
School of Nursing
Vanderbilt University
Nashville, Tennessee

Joanne M. Pohl, PhD, RN, CS, FAAN
Associate Professor
Associate Dean for Community Partnerships
School of Nursing
University of Michigan
Ann Arbor, Michigan

Joseph Purnell
Executive Director
Neighborhood United Against Drugs
Philadelphia, Pennsylvania

The Honorable Marjorie O. Rendell
U.S. Court of Appeals for the 3rd Circuit
Philadelphia, Pennsylvania
Trustee
University of Pennsylvania
Chair
Board of Overseers
School of Nursing
University of Pennsylvania
Philadelphia, Pennsylvania

Hila Richardson, RN, DrPH, FAAN
Professor and Director of Undergraduate Studies
Continuing Education and Community Partnerships
Division of Nursing
New York University
New York, New York

Nancy L. Rothman, EdD, RN
Independence Professor of Community Nursing
Department of Nursing
Temple University
College of Allied Health Professions
Philadelphia, Pennsylvania

Juliann G. Sebastian, PhD, ARNP, FAAN
Professor
Assistant Dean for Advanced Practice Nursing
MSN and Post-MSN Programs
Co-director
DNP Program, College of Nursing
University of Kentucky
Lexington, Kentucky

Diane L. Spatz, PhD, RN
Assistant Professor of Health Care of Women and Childbearing Nursing
School of Nursing
University of Pennsylvania
Philadelphia, Pennsylvania

Marcia Stanhope, DSN, RN, FAAN
Good Samaritan Professor and Chair in Community Health Nursing
Associate Dean
College of Nursing
University of Kentucky
Lexington, Kentucky

Marilyn Stringer, PhD, CRNP
Associate Professor of Women's Health Nursing
School of Nursing
University of Pennsylvania
Philadelphia, Pennsylvania

Neville E. Strumpf, PhD, RN, FAAN
Edith Clemmer Steinbright Professor in Gerontology
Director of the Center for Gerontologic Nursing Science
School of Nursing
University of Pennsylvania
Philadelphia, Pennsylvania

Eileen Sullivan-Marx, PhD, CRNP, FAAN, RN
Associate Professor of Nursing
School of Nursing
University of Pennsylvania
Philadelphia, Pennsylvania

Beth Ann Swan, PhDC, CRNP
Adjunct Assistant Professor
Special Projects Coordinator
Former Associate Director for Operations
Penn Nursing Network (PNN)
School of Nursing
University of Pennsylvania
Philadelphia Pennsylvania

Carolyn A. Williams, PhD, RN, FAAN
Professor and Dean
College of Nursing
University of Kentucky
Lexington, Kentucky

M. Dee Williams, PhD, RN
Professor and Executive Associate Dean and Associate Dean for Clinical Affairs
University of Florida College of Nursing
Gainesville, Florida

Preface

Lois K. Evans and Norma M. Lang

Recognition of the importance of clinical practice to schools of nursing has accelerated over the past several decades. Deans and faculty have tried a range of models to enhance opportunities to make practice an essential component of their school's mission—right alongside of education and scholarship. Examples include the unification model, partnerships with health institutions, faculty practice plans, nurse-managed centers, joint appointments, clinical appointments, joint practices, and collaborative practice arrangements. We conceptualized this book with the conviction that a collection of chapters describing a decade of work—1992 to 2002—to integrate the education, research, and practice components of the mission of a school of nursing would be useful to others. We chose to title the book *Academic Nursing Practice: Helping to Shape the Future of Healthcare* because of our intense belief that nursing holds many of the solutions to the access, quality, and cost problems facing healthcare systems today.

In the five chapters of Part I, we define academic nursing practice and lay out the vision held in the early 1990s—based on a long history—for its promise as an integral component of the tripartite mission of research, education, and practice. Strategic implications for a range of academic practice models are described, together with the importance of strategic planning to guide successful academic practice initiatives. We use our own experience at the University of Pennsylvania School of Nursing to illuminate challenges related to retrofitting practice into a research-intensive institution. Part II focuses in more detail on some of the strategic resources that contribute to academic nursing practice success. Seven of these chapters describe business expertise, financial support and visibility, infrastructure, information systems, resources for integrating research and practice, clinician-educators whose research-practice interface exemplifies the evidence-base building work of faculty in practice, community-academic partnerships that support the tripartite mission, and strategic alliances as a survival strategy. The final chapter describes the contribution of the Penn Macy Initiative for Advancing Academic Nursing Practice to building a critical mass of leaders.

The contributors speak from the vantage point of their own experience, primarily that of the University of Pennsylvania School of Nursing (UPSON), but also that of the schools participating in the Penn Macy Initiative, each of which has been engaged in its own unique academic practice journey over the past decade. In several chapters, Exemplars are included that serve as case examples to highlight major points made in the chapter itself.

It takes 'more than a village' to create and sustain academic nursing practices in research-intensive and other schools of nursing. The most recent success of the movement toward a mature academic practice agenda for nursing is due to the contributions of many people and groups. In particular, we acknowledge

- The faculty and staff of the clinical practices in research- intensive schools of nursing who made the ideas and models of clinical practice actually happen.
- The deans, administrators, and staff of the universities and schools who believed that academic nursing practice would enhance science, learning, and patient care and who acted on that belief by increasing their involvement even to the point of owning, operating, and taking full risk for nursing practices.
- The boards, volunteers, and individual, corporate, and foundation donors who share their expertise and financial support.
- Our community partners, who keep us real and make all the effort worthwhile.
- The Josiah Jr. Foundation and its president, Dr. June Osbourne, who saw the merit of investing in academic practice, thus creating the Penn Macy Initiative.
- The Philadelphia-based Independence Foundation and its president, Susan Sherman, who has sustained a major commitment to the community nursing center model.
- The American Association of Colleges of Nursing, especially Dr. Anne Rhome, who participated in selection, teaching, and bridging for the Penn Macy Initiative, and the faculty and staff teams from 22 research-

intensive university schools of nursing who came to study, learn, and share together at the University of Pennsylvania.

- The Division of Nursing of the U.S. DHHS Health Resources Services Administration for its start-up support for many universities, including UPSON, to develop academic practices, especially nursing centers.
- All of the contributors to this book—chapter and exemplar authors— who were very willing to share their beliefs, experiences, and conceptualizations.

A very special thank you goes to

- Vivian Piasecki, and the honorable Marjorie O. Rendell, for championing academic practice.
- Jennifer Conway, for her brilliant, enthusiastic, and sustained editorial writing support from the first to the last word.
- Lenore Wilkas, supersleuth, for locating and verifying even the most obscure references.
- Tom Gilmore, for his constant support and superb consultation on organizational, political, and futuristic ideas.
- Janet Tomcavage and Kathleen Burke, for their creative management of the Penn Macy Intensive Summer Institutes and follow-up conferences along with their unwaivering commitment to the entire Penn Macy Initiative to Advance Academic Nursing Practice.

Throughout the decade of work, we invoked the oft-quoted notion of Margaret Mead (1999): "Never doubt that a small group of thoughtful committed people can change the world. Indeed, it's the only thing that ever has." Our challenge as a *community-of-interest in the future-of-nursing* is to unite passion and knowledge with the stream of opportunities that emerge—which are frequently out of one's presence and beyond one's control: the economy, demography, new technologies (such as the Internet), and so on. Creating plausible, interesting stories about the future (Gilmore & Shea, 1997) will change the way one looks at the opportunities. These new perceptions will, in turn, produce a readiness to advance and modify ideas that can capitalize on often unpredictable entry points for significant change.

It is the hope of the editors and authors that this book will help— conceptually and practically—others who have a vision of improving healthcare through academic practice. We invite you to help create the next decade of progress and to invent for yourselves the story that you will want to tell in 2014.

REFERENCES

Gilmore, T. N., & Shea, G. P. (1997). Organizational learning and the leadership skill of time travel. *Journal of Management Development, 16*(4), 302–311.
Mead, M. (1999). *Continuities in cultural evolution.* (Originally published 1964.) Piscataway, NJ: Transaction Books.

Part I

The Mission of Academic Nursing Practice: Melding Research, Education, and Clinical Care

Chapter 1

A Vision and a Plan for Academic Nursing Practice

Norma M. Lang and Lois K. Evans

The decade of the 1990s was a time for dreaming and for strategizing ways to realize those dreams. So much appeared to be in place, or nearly in place, that could thrust nursing from the margin into the mainstream. Academic nursing had steadily gained increasing access to federal and philanthropic support for research and demonstration projects. Schools of nursing were increasing their doctorally prepared faculty—many of them advanced practice nurses—who were well-equipped to conduct research, contribute to scholarly development of the discipline, participate in expert clinical practice, and implement evidence-based health care. A steady flow of research findings regarding the superior outcomes of advanced practice nursing care was being produced by university schools of nursing. For the first time, advanced practice nurses (including credentialed faculty) were to gain widespread access to common reimbursement streams for their practice. All this while America was being turned on its ear by the aftermath of major federal efforts to reform health care. And there was a mushrooming managed-care industry and heightened public concerns regarding the persistent erosion of quality of health care. The intersection of these two forces—the strengthening position of nursing and rapidly changing health care policy and delivery environments—was ripe for nursing leadership. How to harness these energies and resources to facilitate change was the question. From the perspective of the academic community, reconfiguring the academic nursing practice paradigm to form an exciting laboratory for change was perceived as one important solution.

Nursing is a practice discipline. Thus, it is not surprising that when nursing is part of an academic institution, faculty and students strive toward the improvement of health care. Academic nursing practice—as a living laboratory that joins actual practice, education, and research—is critical in achieving the missions of schools of nursing, evolving the discipline of nursing, and shaping the future of health care. Where better to demonstrate the efficacy of new practice models and interventions, identify questions for further study, and teach practitioners and research students to think futuristically in their pursuit and application of new knowledge?

Yet, historically, academic nursing had never taken up the challenge of ownership or management of clinical practice to any great degree. Reasons abound as to why this had been so. Fortunately, the period from the 1990s through the turn of the century brought new opportunities for nursing to reclaim—and profoundly change—the practice roots of its social contract. In this chapter, academic nursing practice is defined and the evolution of an expanded paradigm is traced briefly within a historical and sociopolitical context. Readiness factors for academic nursing practice, and the environments and organizational contexts that shape it, are explicated as they relate to further development of a school's practice mission. Associated opportunities and challenges, together with potential solutions, are described for schools of nursing, especially those in an academic health-science center and/or a research-intensive environment. Finally, these points are exemplified through a conceptual description of the structure of academic practice at the University of Pennsylvania School of Nursing (UPSON).

ACADEMIC NURSING PRACTICE: IN SEARCH OF AN EXPANDED PARADIGM

Notions of academic nursing practice have emerged over time with various labels, definitions, and structures and a range of influences on nursing and health care. At the simplest level, academic practices refer to those clinical, administrative, or consultative services associated with university schools of nursing. Since the separation that occurred when nursing education moved from the service setting into institutions of higher education, many mechanisms have been employed to bridge the resulting practice-academy chasm.

What Is Academic Nursing Practice?

Academic nursing practice can be described as "the intentional integration of education, research, and clinical care in an academic setting for the purpose of advancing the science and shaping the structure and quality of health care" (Lang, Evans, & Swan, 2002, p. 63). Key concepts imbedded in this definition include that the integration is deliberate and that it is aimed not only at providing quality evidence-based care but also at educating the next generation of health care professionals and contributing to the development of nursing knowledge and improvement of health care delivery. Through practice associated with a university school of nursing, the components of a tripartite mission can converge, leveraging one through another for greater overall outcomes.

It has been argued that the paradigm "academic nursing practice" goes beyond understandings of "faculty practice" (Evans, Jenkins, & Buhler-Wilkerson, 2003). In the common conception of faculty practice, the individual faculty member is expected to "do" the integration of the tripartite mission in his/her own practice site. While this is a laudable goal, it is seldom satisfactorily achieved without essential infrastructure, built-in supports, and overall mission commitment. Role overload and burnout frequently result (Walker, 1995; Rudy, 2001). In the academic nursing practice paradigm, however, the goals related to practice are themselves integrated within the school's global purpose and vision. A school committed to an academic practice agenda evaluates every new opportunity for its potential to further the overall tripartite mission. Faculty members, individually, may be more or less engaged in specific aspects of the mission, yet, taken together—at the school level—outcomes of integration are achieved. Thus, the whole truly becomes more than the sum of its parts.

Value Added by Academic Nursing Practice

University schools of nursing have a universal commitment to preparing competent practitioners at both beginning and advanced levels of practice (American Association of Colleges of Nursing [AACN], 2000, 1997; Division of Nursing, 2002). Most schools value faculty engagement in scholarly activities ranging from highly funded major programs of research to scholarly applications of teaching and clinical practice (AACN, 1999a, 1999b, 1999c). These two mission functions are more often highly integrated. How practice, however, is integrated within a school of nursing varies widely. For many schools, practice is limited to the use of clinical sites in community health care institutions for student clinical learning experiences. In contrast, for several decades, many university schools of nursing have been engaged in systematically rebuilding closer ties to clinical practice. These relationships are manifest through a variety of arrangements, from the unified ownership/management and partnership models found in academic medical and health centers to faculty practice plans wherein faculty hold appointments in clinical agencies and practicing nurses hold clinical faculty appointments in schools of nursing (see also Chapters 3, 5, & 10 of the present volume; Barger & Rosenfeld, 1993; Christman, 1990; Fehring, Schulte, & Riesch, 1986; Ford, 1980; Ford, 1990; Ford & Kitzman, 1983; Lang, 1983; Lynaugh, Mezey, Aiken, & Buck, Jr., 1984; Riesch, 1992; Sovie, 1989). Although the critically important involvement of competent practitioners in the teaching of students may be assured through these older, well-developed models, less formalized attention has generally been paid to the systematic integration of the research mission. Over the past two decades, increasing numbers of schools of nursing have also engaged in the provision of clinical care through practice(s) that they own, operate, and control, including community-based nurse-managed health centers. In these practices, an explicit intention to blend the three missions is often declared.

Most would agree that academic practice holds great promise and potential for the future of the nursing discipline. Academic nursing practices are living laboratories in which the best evidence-based practice available is delivered, new models are being demonstrated and tested, and access to experience with the business of nursing and health care is assured. This ensures that nursing will have a legitimate place at the table with other disciplines, health care administrators, health care payers, and policy makers. Academic nursing practices offer a community service and an opportunity for community partnerships (see Chapter 11). Educating the next generation of nursing practitioners and leaders requires access to clinical learning laboratories that demonstrate the "possible" for the future of health care (Barger, 1991; Barger & Crumpton, 1991; Conway-Welch & Harshman-Green, 1995; Cotroneo, Outlaw, King, & Brince, 1997; Dreher, Everett, & Hartwig, 2001; Evans, Yurkow, & Siegler, 1994; Lang, Sullivan-

Marx, & Jenkins, 1996; Marek, Jenkins, Westra, & McGinley, 1998; Naylor & Buhler-Wilkerson, 1999).

Conducting clinical research and testing new service models requires a degree of control over the practice setting not often enjoyed by schools of nursing through historically common affiliation arrangements. Given the basic mission of universities—to discover and disseminate knowledge for the betterment of society—academic practice can be said to play a critical role for professional practice schools. Indeed, the other health sciences—medicine, dentistry, veterinary medicine—have operated within a framework of academic practice for much of the last century or longer. Such arrangements have contributed to their research productivity and also to the bottom line in terms of clinical revenue (Burondess, 1991; Krakower, Coble, Williams, & Jones, 2000).

Thus, the vision of an expanded academic nursing practice paradigm has been growing. Academic practice can meet several agendas for schools of nursing and actually serve as the locus for mission integration, all the while making major contributions to the discipline and the health care system. In this vision, academic nursing practice becomes the medium for several important and interlocking agendas. These include testing innovative models of health care delivery; generating new knowledge and implementing the findings from faculty research; developing a common language to measure problems, interventions and outcomes, especially for those addressed by nurses; developing, testing, and implementing evidence-based or best practices; maintaining faculty clinical skills and certification; preparing the next generation of health care leaders, and, generating practice revenue (Evans, Jenkins, & Buhler-Wilkerson, 2003; Lang, Jenkins, Evans, & Matthews, 1996; Walker, 1994; Grey & Walker, 1998; see also Chapter 3). Ultimately, the outcomes of any combination of these agendas can make a major impact. Schools of nursing are increasingly recognizing that innovative integration of such aims is a critical factor in retaining preeminence.

The "why academic nursing practice now" question can be answered in terms of the opportunities afforded by newfound access to practice reimbursement, increasing numbers of faculty with doctoral degrees who are prepared for research *and* advanced practice, the current attention at the national level on nursing practice and its impact on health and mortality outcomes, and the critical state of health care in the nation (Aiken, Clarke, Sloane, Sochalski, & Silber, 2002). What better time than now to capitalize on such profound opportunities? *Carpe diem*, indeed, especially if the school's critical readiness factors are present.

Historical and Socio-political Contexts

With a trajectory different from that of modern medicine, the association between schools of nursing, practice, and health care institutions is one that has changed over time, ranging from a point where all education of nurses occurred in hospitals, to partnerships between schools and hospitals, to schools having only selected student clinical experience in hospitals. In Chapter 2, Lynaugh writes a provocative description of the changing history of nursing education and the practice mission of schools of nursing.

Nursing schools have had limited success in developing and accessing resources similar to those of schools of medicine. Physician and basic scientist faculty in medical schools routinely teach only a few hours a semester, with clinical training of medical students increasingly turned over to residents and interns (Barchi & Lowery, 2000; Levinson & Reubenstein, 1999). In large numbers, physician faculties are engaged in the pursuit of new knowledge and/or clinical practice. Nursing faculty, a comparatively small group in proportion to medical faculty and to the numbers of nursing students, teach many hours a week and can access few, if any, dollars for patient care services. Neither is Graduate Medical Education (GME) support available to most nursing schools or faculty in university schools of nursing (Aiken & Gwyther, 1995).

Whereas academic medicine benefited early on from state and federal regulations that enabled physician faculty to receive payment for practice and also from credentials at the doctoral level that enabled them to secure large research federal dollars, nursing faculty have had access to relatively small amounts of federal and philanthropic support for training and research, and even that has existed only since the 1960s. Most nursing faculty members are salaried by schools, and most school revenues come from state support, tuition, and grants.

A critical mass of nursing faculty with doctorates in some university schools of nursing began to emerge in the 1980s; these faculty members began competing successfully for federal research dollars. Only a small proportion of nursing schools actually receive federal research support; however; schools generally grew because of student numbers, not because of a growth in research funding or practice incomes. Thus, while modest governmental funding for education and research continued, there was and is insufficient support overall for the practice, education and research missions in schools of nursing (Evans, Jenkins, & Buhler-Wilkerson, 2003; see also Chapter 2). In the decade of the 1990s the question arose: Could academic nursing practice not only leverage research and teaching missions but also gain reimbursement and financing for the services provided?

If so, academic nursing practice would not only enrich overall mission achievement but add to revenue as well.

Cautionary Views of Academic Nursing Practice

The verdict is not yet in as to whether mounting an academic practice initiative should be a goal for every school of nursing. Schools that are part of academic medical or health sciences centers may perhaps be better positioned for academic nursing practice because of university commitment to clinical services and access to health care infrastructure support. Schools in research-intensive environments, however, have the depth of scholarship, richness of faculty resources, and leadership potential to best utilize academic practice to move the discipline forward. Thus, these schools, especially, have a greater obligation to address the integration question.

Taking into account these historical contexts, the rationale for deepening the commitment to and/or expanding the paradigm for academic practice on the part of schools of nursing should be examined critically. Academic nursing practice not only provides opportunities but also presents challenges for deans, faculty and university administrators as they plan, strategize, and implement the tripartite mission of research, education and practice. Undertaking academic nursing practice initiatives is not for the faint at heart, especially because of the financial and political risks and time commitments. Regardless of possible positive outcomes, there are those who will, wisely, advocate caution when a school considers investing its scarce resources in a not easily controlled environment—that is, health care systems and financing. The level of financial risk required for owning and operating academic clinical practices, especially for a (usually) small enterprise like a school of nursing, may be greater than is prudent to bear (see Chapter 3). On the other hand, few university administrators and faculty are concerned about small or individual contract practices for which the school has little risk. From the perspective of the university, where the primary mission is education and generating new knowledge, expectations for faculty clinical practice productivity in the current health care environment may be counterproductive to scholarly goals (Barchi & Lowery, 2000).

ORGANIZATIONAL CONTEXTS SHAPING ACADEMIC NURSING PRACTICE

In every school, the evolution of academic nursing practice will be uniquely shaped by its own history, mission and values, and resources and those of its parent university. Further, its geographic, jurisdictional and temporal locations play an important role. Leadership for interpreting the academic practice vision, developing long range/strategic plans, and managing and navigating internal and external environments/contexts and climates, including financial viability, is essential.

History of the School

Understanding the role a school's unique history may play in any new undertaking is important to strategic planning. Previous experiences with clinical practice initiatives in the school, as well as other units of the university (medicine, dentistry, social work, and veterinary medicine) help to shape perceptions of what is possible in the present. How has the university typically measured its overall success and the success of the professional schools? For example, in addition to quality indicators and benchmarks related to numbers and quality of students, placements of graduates, research funding, rankings and national reputations for the university, its schools, and faculty, has the university placed a value on practice or integrated missions? How have practice responsibilities of individual faculty historically been measured and rewarded? Will the expansion of the practice mission require an entirely new paradigm for the university and the school? Chapters 2 and 4 provide additional insights into the impact of historic context and the process of strategic planning.

Mission, Vision, and Values

Mission and vision express the values and serve as explicit statements of the essence of an organization, in this case, the university and the school of nursing. Mission also identifies direction and areas for which resources will be committed. As one embarks on a journey of academic nursing practice development, several questions are well worth examining: Where does academic practice fit in the mission and the vision of the school? Where does academic practice fit in the school's strategic, financial, and operational plans? How does the academic practice focus fit with the mission of the university itself, especially if a research-intensive university? Do the university criteria that are used to measure the success of the school and the faculty include practice?

A review of published mission and vision statements for schools of nursing reveals a range of levels of commitment to practice. For example, UPSON'S mission statement says that

> The mission . . . is to develop, disseminate, and utilize nursing knowledge. Education and *clinical practice* are essential to the utilization of nursing knowledge and generation of questions that give focus and meaning to the research enterprise. Research, education, and *clinical practice* are integrated to create a unique academic milieu in which faculty, clinicians, and students engage in the culture of discovery. [UPSON, 1995; italics added].

In contrast, the role of clinical practice is not as explicit in mission statements such as the following:

- " . . . integrating knowledge development, knowledge transmission, and knowledge application to advance nursing and health care."
- " . . . committed to research and scholarly activity that contributes to the discipline of nursing, and excels in the development, application, and dissemination of knowledge to promote health and well-being for people of the communities, the state, that nation and the world through teaching, research and public service."

Universities and schools of nursing, especially those in land-grant universities, often identify service as a part of their mission statements. Service is usually defined to include university, professional, and community activities of the faculty. Occasionally, service may also include practice activities. In this context—practice as a community (or public) service—revenue generation may or may not be expected. When the academic practice component of the mission is defined and clearly articulated, faculty and administration may have less difficulty garnering commitment of resources—money, time, expertise, and development—for these initiatives.

Readiness Factors for Expanding the Academic Practice Mission

Schools deciding to move beyond affiliations and individual or group faculty practices associated with other health care organizations begin to ask, Is it possible for the school of nursing to own and operate its own practices? If so, what practices, and how will they be organized, operated, quality-controlled, capitalized, and then sustained financially? (A more detailed description of a strategic planning process is found in Chapter 4.)

Readiness Factors

For schools in which the administration and faculty make a commitment to an integrated education, research, and practice mission, the following are factors to be considered as a basis for decision making regarding the expansion of academic nursing practices.

- *Mission*

  ✓ Practice is clearly a central component of the mission of the school
  ✓ Practice is compatible with the university's mission

- *People Resources*

  ✓ A critical mass exists of doctorally prepared faculty and staff to advance all parts of the school's mission
  ✓ A critical mass exists of doctorally prepared faculty with advanced practice expertise
  ✓ A critical mass of advanced practice nurses is available for operating school-owned practices

- *Educational Resources*

  ✓ The School has strong advanced practice and administrative graduate educational programs

- *Research Resources*

  ✓ The school has a history of continuous research funding
  ✓ The school has strong research centers/programs

- *Organizational Resources*

  ✓ There is clear university and school administrative support
  ✓ Sources for financial capital, including fundraising, have been identified

✓ Strong infrastructure staff for the development of business plans, marketing, financial management, and operations are already in place or at least in the plan

✓ Volunteer board members and experts to complement the skills of the school's administration and faculty are available

Each school will need to tailor this list of readiness factors to suit their own environments, both that of the school and of the university.

Geographical, Jurisdictional, and Temporal Assets and Constraints. An assessment of the external environment is also essential in determining readiness for academic practice expansion (Evans, Swan, & Lang, 1993). Rural-urban location will of necessity shape any configuration of an academic practice portfolio. Likewise, richness of current health care offerings in the region, any gaps in services to unserved or underserved groups, degree of managed care penetration, and so on each will have a significant impact.

State practice laws governing the practice of advanced practice nurses, as well as regulations and definitions of such terms as primary care provider, can play major constraining or facilitating roles. The few remaining jurisdictions that restrict or deny privileges for advanced practice nurses, for example, make it much more difficult to construct nurse-managed practices.

Finally, timing often trumps everything! Having a plan for a school-based practice ready to launch just in time for planned major changes in the school district, or an evidence-based intervention developed just when an HMO is ready to implement preventive services to a vulnerable group, or being just behind versus *on* the crest of the wave (when the idea will not be so new as to raise all the original objections) are all important factors to consider. The UPSON experience in expanding its practice mission can be used to exemplify some of these points.

Expanding the Practice Mission at UPSON. By the late 1980s and early 1990s, UPSON had achieved excellence in undergraduate and graduate education and in funded programs of research. There was also a history of strong practice partnerships with the Hospital of the University of Pennsylvania, the Children's Hospital of Philadelphia, and the Visiting Nurse Association of Greater Philadelphia. Clinician-educator faculty held joint appointments in many of these organizations, where they engaged in scholarly practice and leadership (Fagin, 1986). The faculty was generating several new ideas for the further development of practices that were ripe for implementation. Was the school ready to take on the accountability for owning and operating selected practices? Would such a venture enhance the position of UPSON as a national leader in academic nursing practice in research-intensive universities, including clinical scholarship and advanced nursing practice for the next generation of nurses?

The administration, faculty, and volunteer leaders of UPSON believed that these questions could be answered in the affirmative. It was also believed that the readiness factors identified above, including internal and external environmental contexts, had been sufficiently addressed. An intense strategic and long range planning process, aided by expert consultants, resulted in a decision to move forward with redefining the paradigm of academic practice. Over the next decade, the school took full financial risk for creating, owning, and operating selected community-based clinical practices. Midway in that process, in 1995, the school formalized its expanded mission with the creation of the Penn Nursing Network (PNN), an umbrella structure for the school's owned practices. Thus, PNN represented the school's first major venture into full-risk status. PNN's goals were, and are, to build substantial and flexible practice initiatives around faculty strengths as they relate to market opportunities. A more detailed description of PNN is found elsewhere (See Chapters 4, 5, 7, & 8; Evans, Jenkins, & Buhler-Wilkerson, 2003; and Lang, Jenkins, Evans, & Matthews, 1996).

PNN grew to provide best practice models of community-based family-focused health care services to people of all ages in a variety of settings in neighborhoods contiguous to the university campus. With particular attention to the needs of vulnerable populations, advanced practice nursing services have included well-child care, preteen and adolescent care, family planning, women's health, primary care for children and adults, mental health, continence, gerontologic consultation and comprehensive rehabilitation, and integrated acute and long-term care for frail elders. All PNN practices are ambulatory, with appropriate links to specialist consultants and acute and long-term care. While all are school owned and nurse managed, each PNN practice also uniquely demonstrates a model of collaboration with physicians and other health care providers. PNN is intended to function as a vehicle for integrating practice, education, and research. Undergraduate and graduate students whose clinical experiences and preceptorships are in PNN practices have the opportunity to experience firsthand APN-managed models of nursing practice. Practices of PNN also provide a natural laboratory for developing information systems that can be used to measure outcomes of care (See Chapter 8). Such data have significant implications for health policy into the twenty-first century.

UPSON's PNN is among the early innovations nationally that merged the three legs of the stool—education, research and practice—to create an owned and operated component of academic nursing practice. Only a few other schools have tried to cluster such a large number of diverse nursing practices together in a network (See Chapters 3 & 5). The establishment of PNN helped advance the notion that one important way for a school of nursing to enhance innovative evidence-based clinical practice was through controlling the models of care to be implemented and deciding on the mix of different types of nurses and other providers for services. The PNN construct also allowed faculty to collect and control access to the clinical and administrative data that identify the nursing assessments and interventions that produce cost-effective outcomes. Community-based practices of PNN, together with the School's affiliations and partnerships—with the University of Pennsylvania Health System, Children's Hospital of Philadelphia, and the Visiting Nurse Association of Greater Philadelphia (facilitated especially by clinician-educator faculty appointments)—provide access to an even broader range of clinical services from primary care practice to quaternary care. Forging linkages for integrating research in each of these through creative and systematic efforts remains an important goal (see Chapters 9, 10, & 12).

CHALLENGES AND SOLUTIONS

Visions of academic nursing practice can be very clear. Strategic plans can be in place. Good decisions can be made with the best available data. Still, some practices will flourish and some will also decline. The U.S. health care system and market have become more volatile with each passing year. Yet, care needs remain unmet for the many people with chronic health problems; the uninsured; high-risk pregnant women; and those suffering infectious diseases, mental health problems and disorders, and disabilities common in aging. The challenge is to match solutions/care provided by nurses to the needs of people within the fluctuating health care and payment systems. Simultaneously, schools of nursing are faced with the challenges of student enrollments and levels of research support that wax and wane. Demands on faculty for research and teaching productivity are great. A school may not be able to tolerate at a given point in time the added and considerable stress that comes with owning and operating practices.

For schools of nursing, most of which are limited in size and resources, prudence in building an academic practice agenda might prevent overextending faculty and financial resources. Looking for opportunities to add value through partnerships with health care systems and practices, developing clear exit strategies from the start (see Chapter 4), and securing alternate funding streams so as not to rely totally on health care reimbursement are all important strategies to consider (Barchi, 2000). Continually assessing market and environment, regularly collecting and analyzing data on existing practices, surveying current faculty expertise and interests, preparing proposals for future practices, and raising funds through development strategies can help achieve goals. Schools at, for example, the University of Pennsylvania the University of Michigan, and Vanderbilt University, often sought governmental and foundation grants to start practices and then used those dollars to leverage reimbursement from patient revenue sources (See chapter 6 and Exemplars in Chapters 3 & 4).

Administrative, faculty, staff, and volunteer leadership are the keys to making the tripartite mission work. Within an academic enterprise, much planning and discussion occurs before implementing a new educational or research program. The mission and vision for practice require a similar process. When specific practices are under consideration, however, a lengthy process may be deadly to a practice program because of the rapidly changing health care environment. Nimble and flexible are the operative words used to predict success in the health care delivery system. Ideas and business plans must be developed rapidly in response to opportunities. Timely decisions to close a practice must be made as well.

Nursing practices operate in a health care business milieu and require a structure that will accommodate their sensible management. On the other hand, the data from demonstrations and research programs involving practices lose all credibility if programs are changed midstream. This creates potential conflict between the practice sustainability goal and the scholarly goal (see Chapters 4 & 9). Another natural tension is that of faculty time and energy. Will time spent in practice decease teaching and research outputs? Or can a synergy between practice, teaching, and research be developed that creates even better use of time and greater achievements? These potentially opposing forces create identifiable tensions in decision-making. While not espousing a divorce from clinical practice for practice professions, Barchi and Lowery (2000) do suggest a more prudent use of adjunct, clinical, and practice professors rather than assigning heavy practice obligations to tenure track and clinician-educator faculty who should be engaged in scholarly pursuits.

Outside of the traditional medical school and center structure, universities and their administrative units are not experienced in operating, or in assisting schools of nursing to operate, clinical practices. Thus, a question arises: Are there other organizational models that could be pursued, such as a separate corporation outside the university or legal partnerships that share risk? Balancing costly infrastructure requirements (see Chapter 7) with desire for control over model, quality, and access for education and research needs to be negotiated thoughtfully.

An expanded paradigm for academic nursing practice is on the horizon. Many schools have already begun to test its boundaries, refitting its size to their own missions and organizational contexts (see Chapter 13). Those schools that succeed in understanding the importance of their own history, mission, values, and resources and that are skillful in managing external and internal environments will shape nursing for generations to come. In this book, the shared experiences, knowledge, and lessons learned from among those engaged in understanding, testing, and changing academic nursing practice—the University of Pennsylvania and Fellows in the Penn Macy Initiative to Advance Academic Nursing Practice—are offered to help facilitate this journey for many more schools of nursing over the next decade.

REFERENCES

Aiken, L. H., & Fwyther, M. E. (1995). Medicare funding of nurse education: The case for policy change. *JAMA, 273*(19), 1528–1532.

Aiken, L. H., Clarke, S. P., Sloane, D. M., Sochalski, J., & Silber, J. H. (2002). Hospital nurse staffing and patient mortality, nurse burnout, and job dissatisfaction. *JAMA, 288*, 1987–1993.

American Association of Colleges of Nursing (2000). *The baccalaureate degree in nursing as minimal preparation for professional practice* (revised ed). Washington, DC: Author.

American Association of Colleges of Nursing (1999a). *Nursing education's agenda for the 21st century* (revised ed.). Washington, DC: Author.

American Association of Colleges of Nursing (1999b). *Defining scholarship for the discipline of nursing.* Washington, DC: Author.

American Association of Colleges of Nursing (1999c). *Position statement on nursing research* (revised ed.) Washington, DC: Author.

American Association of Colleges of Nursing (1997). *A vision of baccalaureate and graduate nursing education: The next decade.* Washington, DC: Author.

Barchi, R. L. (July 2000). *Academic nursing practice in research-intensive universities: Pros and cons from the provost perspective.* Paper presented at the Penn Macy Initiative to Advance Academic Nursing Practice. Philadelphia: University of Pennsylvania.

Barchi, R. L., & Lowery, B. J. (2000). Scholarship in the medical faculty from the university perspective. *Academic Medicine, 75*(9), 899–905.

Barger, S., & Rosenfeld, P. (1993). Models in community health care: Findings from a National Study of Community Nursing Centers. *Nursing & Health Care, 14,* 426–431.

Barger, S. E. (1991). Entrepreneurial nursing: The right course at the right time. *Nurse Educator, 16*(5), 5–8.

Barger, S. E., & Crumpton, R. B. (1991). Public health nursing partnership: Agencies and academe. *Nurse Educator, 16*(4), 16–18.

Burondess, J. (1991). The academic health center and the public agenda: Whose three-legged stool? *Annals of Internal Medicine, 115,* 962.

Christman, L. (1990). Innovations in nursing education administration. In M. A. Wandelt & B. J. Thomas (Eds.), *Innovations in nursing education administration* (pp. 117–118). New York: National League for Nursing.

Conway-Welch, C., & Harshman-Green, A. (1995). At the table: Nursing in managed care. *Nursing Policy Forum, 1*(5), 10–16.

Cotroneo, M., Outlaw, F. H., King, J., & Brince, J. (1997). Advanced practice psychiatric mental health nursing in a community-based nurse-managed primary care program. *Journal of Psychosocial Nursing, 35*(11), 18–25.

Division of Nursing (2002). *Nurse practitioner primary care competencies in specialty areas: Adult, family, gerontological, pediatric, and women's health.* Washington, DC: Health Resources and Services Administration.

Dreher, M., Everett, L., & Hartwig, S. M. (2001). The University of Iowa Nursing Collaboratory: A partnership for creative education and practice. *Journal of Professional Nursing, 17,* 114–120.

Evans, L. K., Jenkins, M., & Buhler-Wilkerson, K. (2003). Academic nursing practice: Implications for policy. In M. D. Mezey, D. O. McGivern, & E. Sullivan-Marx (Eds.), *Nurse practitioners: Evolution of advanced practice* (4th ed., pp. 443–470). New York: Springer.

Evans, L. K., Yurkow, J., & Siegler, E. L. (1995). The CARE Program: A nurse-managed collaborative outpatient program to improve function of frail older people. *Journal of the American Geriatrics Society, 43,* 1155–1160.

Evans, L. K., Swan, B. A., & Lang, N. M. (2003). Evaluation of the Penn Macy Initiative to Advance Academic Nursing Practice. *Journal of Professional Nursing, 19*(1), 8–16.

Fagin, C. M. (1986). Institutionalizing faculty practice. *Nursing Outlook, 34*(3), 140–144.

Fehring, R. J., Schulte, J., & Riesch, S. K. (1986). Toward a definition of nurse-managed centers. *Journal of Community Health Nursing, 3*(2), 59–67.

Ford, L. C. (1980). Unification of nursing practice, education and research. *International Nursing Review, 27,* 179–183.

Ford, L. C. (1990). A saga in social change: Unification of nursing practice, education, and research. In M. A. Wandelt & B. J. Thomas (Eds.), *Innovations in nursing education administration* (pp. 117–118). New York: National League for Nursing.

Ford, L. C., & Kitzman, H. J. (1983). Organizational perspectives on faculty practice: Issues and challenges. In K.E. Barnard (Ed.), *Structure to outcome: Making it work.*

First Annual Symposium on Nursing Faculty Practice), pp. 13–29). Kansas City, MO: American Nurses Association.

Grey, M., & Walker, P. H. (1998). Practice-based research networks for nursing. *Nursing Outlook, 46,* 125–129.

Krakower, J. Y., Coble, T. Y., Williams, D. J., & Jones, R. F. (2000). Review of U.S. medical school finances, 1998–1999. *JAMA, 284*(9), 1127–1129.

Lang, N. M. (1983). Nurse-managed centers: Will they thrive? *American Journal of Nursing, 13*(9), 1290–1292.

Lang, N. M., Jenkins, M., Evans, L. K., & Matthews, D. (1996). Administrative, financial, and clinical data for an academic nursing practice: A case study of the University of Pennsylvania School of Nursing. In *The power of faculty practice: Proceedings of the American Association of Colleges of Nursing's 1995 and 1996 Faculty Practice Conferences.* Washington, DC: AACN.

Lang, N. M., Sullivan-Marx, E., & Jenkins, M. (1996). Advanced practice nurses and success of organized delivery systems. *American Journal of Managed Care, 2,* 129–135.

Lang, N. M., Evans, L. K., & Swan, B. A. (2002). Penn Macy Initiative to Advance Academic Nursing Practice. *Journal of Professional Nursing, 18*(2), 63–69.

Levinson, W., & Rubenstein, R. (1999). Sounding Board. Mission critical—Integrating clinician-educators into academic medical centers. *The New England Journal of Medicine, 341*(11), 840–843.

Lynaugh, J. E., Mezey, M. D., Aiken, L., & Buck, C. R., Jr. (1984). The teaching nursing home: Bringing together the best. *American Health Care Association Journal, 10*(3), 24–28.

Marek, K. D., Jenkins, M., Westra, B. L., & McGinley, A. (1998). Implementation of a clinical information system in nurse-managed care. *Canadian Journal of Nursing Research, 30,* 37–44.

Naylor, M. D., & Buhler-Wilkerson, K. (1999). Creating community-based care for the new millennium. *Nursing Outlook, 47,* 120–127.

Riesch, S. K. (1992). Nursing centers: An analysis of the anecdotal literature. *Journal of Professional Nursing, 8*(1), 16–25.

Rudy, E. B. (2001). Supportive work environments for nursing faculty. *AACN Clinical Issues, 12*(3), 401–410.

Sovie, M. D. (1989). Clinical nursing practices and patient outcomes: Evaluation, evolution, and revolution: Legitimizing radical change to maximize nurses' time for quality care. *Nursing Economic$, 7*(2), 79–85.

University of Pennsylvania School of Nursing (1995, November). Mission of the School of Nursing. In *Faculty Manual.* Philadelphia: Faculty Senate.

Walker, P. H. (1994). A comprehensive community nursing center model: Maximizing practice income—A challenge to educators. *Journal of Professional Nursing, 10*(3), 131–139.

Walker, P. H. (1995). Faculty practice: Interest, issues, and impact. In J. Fitzpatrick & J. Stevenson (Eds.), *Annual Review of Nursing Research,* pp. 217–235. New York: Springer.

Chapter 2

Academic Nursing Practice: Looking Back

Joan E. Lynaugh

Historians who explore the recent past do so at their peril. Perspective is uncertain, and personal recollections of individuals often conflict with or contradict each other. Moreover, the events under scrutiny are still unfolding, rendering well-documented and well-rounded conclusions impossible. Inevitably, further innovations, changing environments, and new academic problems will importantly alter our future ideas about academic nursing practice. Nevertheless, I am arguing here that our history as nurse educators persistently pervades and influences our ideas and our beliefs about academic nursing practice today. Moreover, the reality of nursing practice, nursing education, and nursing research, the trinity that now constitutes the mission of higher education in nursing, is built on our collective memory. The need to understand where we stand in the historical scheme of things justifies examining our recent history.

First, let us ask ourselves why academic nursing practice continues to pose problems for us, both in concept and in implementation. How did it come to be that nurses found it necessary in the 1970s to remind each other that nursing is a practice profession? Even a superficial look at the history of higher education in nursing gives us the answer.

As early as 1909, a split in the fabric of nursing effectively separated those who nursed the sick from those who taught and studied nursing at the college level. The first college courses in nursing at Teacher's College, Columbia University, in New York City, were not about caring for the sick or how to practice nursing. Those courses, and the education for nurses in other college programs in the first half of the twentieth century, concentrated on preparing supervisors for hospitals, teachers for nursing schools, and administrators for public health and visiting nurse societies. We can find occasional deviations from the norm. For example, Martha Ruth Smith and Virginia Henderson did develop and teach a course on medical surgical asepsis at Teacher's College in 1930. Their classes were based on actual patient care problems and included a clinical component. The course, however, was controversial, depended on their persistence, and remained unique.

The historical record shows that academic nurses' experience with clinical practice is really rather recent, dating back only about 40 or 50 years. Expanding the mission of colleges of nursing so as to include practice as a vital component meant changing everything about those colleges and their faculty. I begin this chapter by outlining a series of historical events in nursing education since World War II, with special emphasis on the last three decades of the twentieth century. This, I hope, will help clarify the complicated environment out of which our present day ideas of academic nursing practice emerged.

Then I will illustrate some issues affecting academic nursing practice by taking an in-depth look at relevant experiments and fundamental changes undertaken at the University of Pennsylvania School of Nursing (UPSON). My belief is that the details of UPSON's story can serve as a useful case study, helping us to gain needed historical perspective on the meaning and merit of academic nursing practice as we move along in the twenty-first century.

NURSING EDUCATION IN THE POST-WORLD WAR II ERA

When World War II ended, Americans, finally convinced of their leadership role in the world and more affluent than at any time in history, turned their attention to domestic problems. High on the list of work to be done were building a larger, better system of higher education and building a larger, better health care system. Nursing found itself at the intersection of these concerns; its future would be markedly affected by local and national decision-making regarding higher education and the expanding health care system.

The G.I. Bill of 1944 proved to be very attractive to returning veterans and virtually guaranteed rapid growth of America's colleges and universities. Then, in 1946, President Harry Truman appointed the President's Commission on Higher Education (usually called the Truman Commission), which advocated universal access to higher education for individuals with interest and ability. Among its many recommendations was expansion of the country's two-year junior colleges. Incidentally, to improve their image as an integral part of the higher education system, junior colleges were renamed community colleges.

True to the aspirations of the Truman Commission, over the next 30 years the number of students enrolled in higher education would grow tenfold, the number of faculty would grow sixfold, and the number of educational institutions would double (Cohen, 1998). Some of those new students, faculty, and institutions would be nurses and nursing schools. When we recall that only about one in four Americans completed high school before World War II, we can better appreciate just how dramatic an educational change was underway by 1950.

Hospital Expansion

At virtually the same time, The Hospital Survey and Reconstruction Act (Hill-Burton), also signed by Harry Truman in 1946, provided money to states and local communities for hospital and other health facility development. Contributions by employers to health insurance as a form of nontaxable wage benefit became common, and health insurance through employment boomed. In 1946, only about one-third of Americans held some form of insurance; by 1960, however, three quarters of Americans held health care insurance that gave them access to hospital and medical care. The combination of expanding hospitals and insured citizens' access to hospital care and medical services created heavy and persistent demand for hospital nurses (Lynaugh & Brush, 1996).

Criticisms of Nursing Education

In the late 1940s, 1,100 hospital schools of nursing educated almost all the nation's nurses. This arrangement did not satisfy nursing's leadership, and it was also increasingly seen as a problem by hospital leaders who complained that maintaining the nursing schools unfairly burdened hospitals with unrecoverable costs. Study after study recommended relocating the education of nurses from hospital-owned schools to colleges and universities. Esther Lucile Brown focused specifically on education as a crucial element in the recurring problems of supply and demand for nurses. She argued that there was something fundamentally wrong with a system of education that could meet neither qualitative nor quantitative requirements for nurses. Brown's 1948 report, *Nursing for the Future*, found wide acceptance in nursing and became the blueprint for an agenda for nursing reform (Brown, 1948).

It was, however, not simply a matter of expanding baccalaureate programs and graduating more nurses with baccalaureate degrees. What confronted nursing deans and faculty was a complete rethinking of the purposes of baccalaureate education and the mission of schools of nursing. Most baccalaureate nursing programs of the 1950s were small. Their students were those graduates of hospital diploma programs who wished to become teachers or nurse administrators or to qualify for positions in public health. At many universities, both baccalaureate and hospital-based diploma programs existed side by side. The diploma program was typically larger and provided the nursing staff for the university hospital. The small number of generic baccalaureate students who had no previous preparation in nursing usually joined the diploma students for three years of clinical courses after completing two years of college. As a result, faculty in baccalaureate schools of nursing rarely were expected to teach content that actually dealt with direct patient care or to clinically supervise student practice. Instruction in direct care of patients was the province of faculty who taught in the diploma programs, or, more commonly, the head nurses and supervisors in the hospitals where students were assigned. College faculty degrees were likely to be in education, public health, or perhaps the social sciences. Few aspired to be clinically competent, and neither was this expected of them.

AGENDA FOR CHANGE

Converting this peculiar educational patchwork to a more coherent system capable of producing an adequate number of well-prepared nurses for direct patient care would occupy and frustrate two generations of postwar nurse leaders and educators. They faced several formidable tasks. First, they needed to find and prepare competent nurse faculty who could qualify for university appointments and actually teach novices how to nurse the sick. They had to negotiate with hospitals, public health agencies, and other clinical sites for learning opportunities for their students, including access to patients. They had to find a way to pay the high costs of clinical education for students. And, they had to convince university and college administrators that schools of nursing could become financially viable.

The federal government, acting through the Division of Nursing of the Public Health Service, became a major force in the effort to improve nursing education. Founded in 1946, the division ultimately became a conduit for statistical information about nursing and for federal funds to address some of the most serious problems in nursing. It began to fund nursing research projects in 1955 at the same time as it was underwriting conferences to educate nurses about research methods. Although the National Mental Health Act supported graduate education in psychiatric nursing as early as 1946, it would be 10 more years before new funds were authorized for general nursing education. The Health Amendments Act of 1956 allocated money to prepare nurses to become teachers, supervisors, and nursing service administrators. This money could be used for baccalaureate education, thus helping to build the tiny pool of degree-holding nurses. It was, however, slow work. By 1965, only one nurse in seven held a college degree.

During the 1960s, federal involvement accelerated. In 1963, the surgeon general of the United States issued the report *Toward Quality in Nursing* (U.S. Surgeon General, 1963) which formally declared the nation's qualitative and quantitative shortage of nurses. Estimating that the number of nurses in the United States needed to triple during the 1960s and that the nation needed four times as many nurses with baccalaureate degrees, the report emphasized federally subsidized loans and scholarships for students. It also called for expanding funds for graduate study and for nursing research. *Toward Quality in Nursing* became the blueprint for a new structure of federal assistance for nursing. In 1964, the Nurse Training Act added Title VIII to the Public Health Service Act; this funding set off an array of nursing initiatives. New buildings for schools of nursing, curricular experimentation, faculty development, and an expanded Professional Nurse Traineeship Program all helped to make relocation of nursing education into higher education a real possibility.

Local changes in nursing education also swept the nation in the 1950s and early 1960s. Beginning in 1952, entirely new programs were created at the county or city level; these were in the tax-supported community colleges recommended by the Truman Commission on Higher Education.

During the next 10 years, 84 new programs opened to educate nurses in community colleges across the country. Gradually, the number of hospital-based diploma programs began to decline as the community college nursing programs continued to grow.

New Knowledge and New Expectations in Nursing

Education of nurses was moving from hospitals to colleges, vastly increased funding from local and federal sources was becoming available to educators, and the numbers of nurses and demand for their services were growing rapidly. A kind of restless and erratic change pervaded nursing during the 1960s and 1970s. Now add exploding biomedical knowledge and new technology applied to treating the sick and preventing illness. Pharmaceuticals such as broad-spectrum antibiotics, diuretics, the thiazides, and new drugs for treating cancer completely revised treatment of infectious disease, heart failure, mental illness, and cancer. Ventilators, monitors, electric beds, disposable equipment, and a bewildering flood of tubes and wires enhanced care and harried health care workers with their complexity.

At least two clinical care realities inherent in this biomedical and technological revolution bore down on nurse educators. First, changes in care were so constant that, to be useful, nursing knowledge had to be conceptual, adaptive, and constantly refreshed. Conservative nursing habits of teaching standard procedures and then expecting learners to adhere carefully to one way of doing things failed in the face of rapid changes in knowledge. Second, some of the most dramatic therapeutic aspects of the so-called biomedical revolution could not be applied to patients' needs unless nurses took responsibility for them.

By the very design of the hospital-focused health and medical care system, the only persons continuously present with the patient were nurses. For example, it quickly became apparent that there was no point in monitoring the heart rhythm of the cardiac patient unless the nurse knew how and when to intervene if an arrthymia occurred (Fairman & Lynaugh, 1998). New understanding of the electrophysiology of the heart and continuous monitoring technology quickly elevated care expectations of nurses. To care safely for patients, nurses needed to know and do more. Success meant they had to act independently on their own science-based knowledge rather than apply poorly fitting standard procedures. Importantly, capable nurses began to be defined and recognized for their ability to incorporate new information into their care and to teach others how to do the same.

Authority in nursing came to rest on clinical ability and not just on the nurse's rank in the hospital hierarchy.

The Spread of Specialization

At the same time, nurses' scope of practice kept expanding into new areas. When knowledge and new applications of knowledge expand rapidly, our modern response is to specialize, thereby dividing up the work into manageable pieces. Exactly that happened in hospital nursing. Of course, for many decades, some nurses practiced in specialized areas; think, for example, of nurse anesthetists, nurse midwives, and public health nurses. During the 1970s, however, the rapid explosion in biomedical knowledge and new treatments for gravely ill patients suffering from chronic illnesses spun off oncology nurses, coronary care and then critical care nurses, nephrology nurses, neonatal nurses, and many more, including primary care nurses. These new specialists joined the clinical specialists in psychiatric–mental health nursing who began practicing in the 1960s.

This segmentation emerged from the banding together of like-minded nurses seeking to improve their practice and safeguard their patients. Newsletters, conferences, manuals, and journals, together with new specialty organizations, began to appear as these self-declared specialists tried to share knowledge to meet the care problems presented by their patients. The media, the meetings, and the organizations were the self-educational efforts of ordinary practicing staff nurses. It would be a decade or more before nurse educators in the nation's colleges could catch up with changing practice in the nation's hospitals.

Responses of Schools of Nursing

The lag in educational response to the changing scene in patient care was caused by two prevailing conditions in nursing education. As noted earlier, most postwar baccalaureate programs focused on preparing diploma school graduates to teach in diploma schools, administer nursing service in hospitals, or work in public health. Most generic students experienced traditional diploma school training as a supplement to their two years of introductory arts and sciences courses. Add to that the scarcity of master's level nurses. For instance, in 1962, just slightly over 1,000 nurses were graduates of master's programs; this represented about 10% of the number that would be recommended by the authors of *Toward Quality in Nursing* (Surgeon General, 1963).

The result was that few schools of nursing in the 1960s were offering either a fully developed college nursing major to undergraduates or producing the necessary potential faculty to rectify the situation. The resulting educational crisis helped stimulate the political will to pay for better education of nurses and inspire private foundations and state governments to join the federal government in supporting reform. In particular, as mentioned earlier, the Nurse Training Act of 1964 offered real impetus to improving college-based education for nurses.

This combined private and public response also helped graduate education for nurses grow rapidly in the 1970s. The pattern of offerings at the master's level began to include specialization in a preferred clinical area as well as preparation in traditional areas of teaching, administration, or research. Then, later in the decade, schools came under pressure to upgrade clinical preparation so that graduates could provide expert care in their area of preparation. Escalating expectations for nursing practice in critical care, oncology, primary care, care of the elderly, and many other areas influenced these programs. Moreover, practicing nurses enrolling in graduate study and armed with funding demanded clinically relevant courses. As the decade drew to a close, graduates of more clinically rich programs began to join the faculties in schools of nursing and continued the trend. Faculty preparing nursing administrators adapted the specialty mode as well. Nursing administration became the main focus of distinct programs instead of a functional minor.

By the late 1970s, and continuing throughout the 1980s and 1990s, the content of nursing curricula and the interest and competence of nursing faculty significantly shifted toward clinical practice. This change in focus was encouraged and enhanced by several well-known and influential experiments in the structure of nursing schools in universities.

EXPERIMENTS TO CLOSE
THE PRACTICE–EDUCATION GAP

Initiatives leading to what we now call academic nursing practice began to appear as early as the 1960s. The integral relationship between practice and learning in a practice-based discipline such as nursing meant that deans and faculty needed to find a way to ensure that faculty were competent to teach clinical nursing. Students could only learn nursing through access to patients. One high cost of moving nursing education out of hospitals was the geographic, psychological, and experiential distance created among teachers, students, and nurses caring for patients. That distance is what I am choosing to call the practice–education gap.

In 1956, Dorothy Smith, an innovative dean determined to address this issue, joined her school of nursing with the new hospital nursing care system at the University of Florida in Gainesville. She brought the care of patients and the education of students under her leadership and applied that "unified" model throughout the system. Among her goals were to demonstrate a high level of intellectual and clinical nursing that would influence people's concept of the nature of nursing, facilitate faculty practice, assemble nursing data, and create nursing systems. For a variety of reasons, including changes in leadership in the university, Smith's experiment failed after about 14 years. Her work was widely acclaimed, however, and other models intended to link education and practice emulated her example.

In 1969, Case Western Reserve University's Frances Payne Bolton School of Nursing, aided by federal funding, launched its Experiment in Nursing. In proposing academic leadership for nursing, the concept empowered faculty to name certain leadership positions in clinical agencies linked with the school. The new University of Rochester School of Nursing opened as a "unified" model in 1972. With funding from the W.K. Kellogg Foundation, the intent was to encourage nurse faculty to accept responsibility for patient care while sustaining their academic teaching and research work, thus, bringing the benefits of their scholarship to bear on patient care. Rush University in Chicago created its own version of a unified model in 1972. Thus, by the 1970s, clinically based curricula and "faculty practice" became something of an academic ideal. In addition to its educational advantages, unifying education and practice also offered nursing schools a way to underwrite some of the costs of education by sharing faculty salaries. Furthermore, faculty access to patients in hospitals and other settings facilitated their ability to develop and carry out clinically focused research.

It would be incorrect, however, to imagine that some panacea for the dilemmas of higher education in nursing was to be found in these examples. Trying to meet higher standards for faculty appointment in colleges and universities, greater demands for more sophisticated course work, and increasing pressures for clinical competence while trying to build nursing research with under-funded budgets ensured that efforts to link academic nursing with the practice of nursing would continue to be difficult.

Moreover, the language employed in discussions about closing the practice–education gap tells us something more about the problem. Collaboration, faculty practice, unification, nursing centers, and academic practice
were just a few of the words and phrases that were used in the sometimes
edgy dialogue between those who cared for patients and those who taught
nurses. As Claire Fagin pointed out in 1986, fruitful connections are about
more than structure (Fagin, 1986).

The language suggests that the people involved in these projects probably
were willing to collaborate or work together. But few were willing or able
to see their nursing territory or responsibility subjugated in the name of
"unification." Academics might philosophize that nursing is a practice
profession and, thus, argue that improvements in clinical practice were
an academic responsibility. Nurse leaders in hospitals and other clinical
agencies, focusing on meeting patient care obligations within budget constraints and on a 24-hour, 7-day-a-week, 365-day-a-year schedule, were
often cool to such faculty aspirations.

One way around the problem of differing objectives between school and
hospital was for the school to open its own care facility. The idea of what
came to be called nursing centers spread rather rapidly during the 1980s.
Perhaps the first modern nursing center was opened in New York City by
Lydia Hall in 1962. The Loeb Center for Nursing and Rehabilitation at
Montefiore Hospital and Medical Center in the Bronx was entirely nurse-
run and offered a wide range of services and programs for people needing
post hospital rehabilitation. Then, during the 1970s and 1980s, small
centers began to appear; many of these, though not all, were connected
with schools of nursing (see Chapter 12).

One motive for schools taking this step sprang from their need for clinical
teaching sites for undergraduate and graduate students. In particular, it
was difficult to find well or moderately ill people with whom students
could work. Patients in hospitals, the typical site for clinical teaching,
were, by this time, seriously ill and not suitable for many types of clinical
experiences. Another reason schools moved in this direction was to set up
demonstration projects for research purposes. Typically, nursing centers
focused on underserved populations. To a certain extent, the movement
was helped along by local and state health initiatives, by interested private
foundations, and by the federal government. A wide variety of people were
served by these centers—ranging from maternity and child care, to care
of the aging, to addiction counseling and social assistance, to screening
programs and primary care.

ACADEMIC PRACTICE AT THE END
OF THE TWENTIETH CENTURY

The effort to bridge the practice–education gap was aided in the last two decades of the twentieth century by growing consensus about the scope of nursing practice. The idea of nurses practicing independently in the community, which seemed aberrant in 1965, aroused less reaction as time went on. Nurses began to be more successful in extracting themselves from the medical oversight of their practice and gradually gained prescribing privileges and other opportunities previously held only by physicians. Moreover, perhaps emboldened by their new sense of clinical capability as nurse practitioners or advanced practice nurses, nurses became less dependent on nursing hierarchies in hospitals or other agencies to guide and protect them.

On the other hand, direct reimbursement for nursing services by third-party payers was difficult to achieve. Not only were nursing services not reimbursed, but the kinds of services nursing centers wanted to provide also were not covered under government or private insurance systems. Educating patients and advocating for social services and many preventive care services were and are not covered by insurance. Finding ways to generate revenue required sophisticated knowledge of a highly complex health care reimbursement system and new financial skills.

In many ways, widespread concern about America's health care system with its rising costs, the problem of under insured and uninsured people, the aging population, the AIDS crisis, and other issues actually helped change the dialogue. When nurses proposed solutions for some of these problems, they found an audience previously denied them.

THIRTY YEARS OF EXPERIMENT AND CHANGE AT THE
UNIVERSITY OF PENNSYLVANIA

As we think of academic nursing practice at UPSON, it is important to remember that nurses have learned and worked on the University of Pennsylvania campus since 1886 when the Board of Women Visitors convinced the trustees that a school of nursing was essential to the success of its hospital. The Hospital of the University of Pennsylvania (HUP), opened in 1874, was the nation's first university-owned hospital. Nevertheless, it suffered from the same seemingly intractable problems as did all nineteenth-century hospitals. Inadequate patient care, bad housekeeping, erratic management, and chronic lack of money all conspired to defeat the institution and endanger its patients. HUP's Nurses Training School solved at least the first three of these problems for the university. Moreover, its leaders and graduates played a significant role in establishing the new profession of nursing at the turn of the twentieth century.

Contentious Change

Forty-nine years after the hospital training school opened, the university's trustees approved a department of nursing in the School of Education. This 1935 decision established the forerunner of the present school. Then, in 1950, the university created a school of nursing, naming Theresa I. Lynch its first dean. Twenty-seven years later, the hospital school was closed. The interval between the founding of UPSON in 1950 and the closure of the hospital diploma program in 1977 was characterized by conflict and acrimony between the two programs.

While some of the conflict was the result of individual loyalty to the longstanding diploma school versus the university program, the heart of the matter rested on perceptions about which graduates could exhibit greater clinical competence and deliver safe patient care. Indeed, the onus was on the university school to demonstrate that its faculty and its graduates could measure up when it came to taking care of patients. Notice that perceptions, not reality or direct comparison of ability, were at issue here. Recall, too, that university schools of nursing, including that of UPSON, were, until that time, mainly turning out teachers and nursing administrators, not clinicians.

It was in this environment that the UPSON faculty of the late 1970s thought about reframing their curricula and redirecting their academic future. Questions about the best relationship with HUP and other needed clinical facilities, about reconfiguration of faculty roles and responsibilities, about new directions for curriculum and research, and about the ever vexing problem of budgeting for essential clinical education and research opportunities crowded the agenda.

Considering the Practice Agenda

In 1975, a new family nurse clinician program at the master's level began to turn out nurses who sought careers as direct caregivers. At UPSON, as was true elsewhere, faculty began to develop more clinically focused and specialty oriented courses. These initiatives did not, however, do anything to solve the problem of access to patients for education and research. In fact, they created an even greater need for better access to a wider array of clinical resources.

Throughout the late 1970s and early 1980s, UPSON's Long Range Planning Committee spent a lot of time on the practice issue. There was much discussion about models for collaboration; the committee discovered that about 10% of the faculty already functioned in combined teaching and practice roles, while many nurse clinicians from the hospital taught students in UPSON's undergraduate and graduate offerings. What was happening was that leaders in midwifery, the nurse practitioner programs, the critical care program, the psychiatric-mental health program, and others recruited and supported clinically active faculty in the various ways needed to teach students in a successful clinical program. Thus, an eclectic approach to what we now call academic nursing practice emerged from the demands of a changing curriculum in which students were being prepared for specialized direct care.

These programmatic initiatives did not happen in a vacuum, of course. As former Dean Claire Fagin wrote in 1986, and, as I have been arguing here, the very idea of the school of nursing was changing. Sometime in the 1970s, the prevailing view of a university school of nursing changed from a place where nursing should be taught and learned to a place where nursing should be taught, learned, *and* practiced (Fagin, 1986).

Vastly complicating the realization of this idea was the equally compelling need and desire to develop nursing scholarship and build a research base at UPSON. The problem the faculty faced was how to understand and implement their new imagination of UPSON. Faculty and clinicians engaged in a very long and somewhat torturous planning process with many starts and stops. Interestingly, the process itself tended to develop shared educational and practice activities as mutual interests in teaching, practice, and research were discovered.

Partnership Efforts

After at least five years of meetings, a joint proposal called Partnership in Nursing was produced in 1984. This draft proposal was roughly based on the idea of unification and included a complex and detailed model to weave the division of nursing at the HUP together with UPSON. The proposed model was deliberately similar to the structure of the medical school. The Partnership proposal included philosophy, organization, governance, and implications for research, education, and practice. It also created a large number of administrative roles and raised some thorny questions of academic autonomy and reporting relationships. The document was widely shared and elicited broad response. Questions of budget control, effect on the nursing staff at HUP, effect on research directions, and implications for relations with clinical entities other than HUP were raised.

In the end, the Partnership In Nursing proposal wound up on the shelf. It was judged to be too focused on unification, too complicated and unwieldy, and unlikely to meet either the broader objectives of the faculty or the clinical goals of nursing in the hospital.

Clinician-Educator Track

While faculty and clinicians worked on the partnership model, a more fruitful but equally lengthy project sought to develop new university appointment options that could be consistent with the interests of nursing faculty who wished to practice. That is, the intent was to redesign the appointment system so that faculty engaged in practice could share all the rights and privileges of the standing faculty of UPSON. The faculty found a precedent for solving this problem in the already existing clinician-educator appointment track in the medical and dental schools. Nursing moved forward with the idea in 1982. Arguing that the future of UPSON depended on developing a research and scholarly base, providing excellent educational programs, and fostering clinical excellence in associated health care settings, the faculty approved a final resolution establishing a clinician-educator track in 1983 (Lowery, 1983).

Faculty accepting these new clinician-educator appointments joined the standing faculty of the University of Pennsylvania on a nontenure track. Qualified faculty were appointed using the regular systems of UPSON with time limits for promotion and requirements for practice carefully spelled out. All income generated by faculty practice reverted to the school while their salaries were consistent with faculty policies. The duration of clinician-educator appointments was linked to the duration of their practice. Some safeguards were set to enable clinician-educators to change practice settings. Limits on the percent of the total faculty who could be clinician-educators were set at 30% of the total faculty (later changed to 40%; see Clinician-Educator Track, 1983). Those limits were intended to allay university faculty fears that the tenure system would be undermined by professional schools' appointing too many faculty outside the tenure system.

The deliberations on the clinician-educator track seemed to clarify the faculty's overall view of how the trinity of research, practice, and teaching might be accomplished. Each nursing faculty member needed to think through the personal implications of focusing on research and publishing. Did this mean they would not have to teach? No. It did mean that being an expert teacher would not be enough to warrant promotion for tenure-track faculty. In importance, research and scholarship moved in from the margins and became central to the school. Did this mean that faculty on the tenure track did not have to be expert clinicians? Yes, it probably did mean that the most expert clinicians would be in the clinician-educator track. At the same time, however, it also meant that expert practice combined with teaching warranted standing faculty status and privileges for clinician educators.

Coming to a Workable Consensus

In the end, three propositions in some sort of balance emerged from the prolonged conversation. First, a nursing faculty needs to work toward the development and dissemination of new knowledge relevant to the profession. Second, a nursing faculty needs to be highly qualified to teach the knowledge and skills necessary to prepare excellent practitioners of the art and science of nursing. And, finally, it did not seem necessary that each faculty member individually embody all three capabilities; in fact, some primarily practice, some primarily do research, and all communicate their work to improve their own knowledge and that of their students (Lowery, 1983).

Certain clinicians, then, sought faculty appointment as clinician-educators with contracted responsibilities at HUP, Children's Hospital of Philadelphia (CHOP), and various other patient care agencies linked to UPSON. At the same time, nurses in practice accepted more limited clinical faculty appointments in the associated faculty according to their teaching responsibilities. Although, over time, a number of memoranda of understanding and other agreements evolved, the faculty practice gap was closed more by individuals linking entities together than by any major structural arrangements. The outcome of all those conversations at UPSON during the 1980s turned out be an academic nursing practice concept based on individual action rather than on organizational restructuring (Fagin, 1986).

By the 1990s, the School of Nursing expressed its mission of research, education, and practice as an integrated whole. The doctoral program was well developed and faculty research well funded and widely acclaimed. Undergraduate and graduate programs attracted high caliber students. In the middle of the decade, under the direction of Dean Norma Lang, UPSON launched the idea of a network of practices to support its tripartite mission. The concept required that new practices needed to have a clear research agenda, provide educational services for undergraduate and graduate students, have an adequate funding stream, and assure safe ongoing care for those it served (UPSON, 1997).

The Penn Nursing Network (PNN), a set of nurse-managed practices, was developed in neighboring communities, many with underserved, vulnerable populations. In effect, PNN complements UPSON's more long-standing links with Penn's hospitals, CHOP, the Visiting Nurse Association of Greater Philadelphia, and other clinical agencies where UPSON students and faculty practice and learn.

Examples of PNN's ambulatory care practices included a day hospital for frail, older adults, a community midwifery practice, a continence program, a gerontologic nursing consultation service, and a primary care practice in a local recreation center. Moreover, UPSON invested in the Program of All-inclusive Care for the Elderly (PACE) called LIFE (Living Independently For Elders), which provides comprehensive care for very dependent older adults living in its neighborhood. PNN's innovation, described elsewhere in more detail, is a logical consequence of three decades of experimentation. The extent to which PNN meets its goals as well as the problems it encounters are, it would seem, reflective of the ideals, reality, and history of academic nursing practice.

THEMES IN ACADEMIC NURSING PRACTICE

I reiterate the assertion I made at the beginning of this chapter; that is, final conclusions on the history of academic nursing practice are impossible at this early stage. Still, some persisting themes do emerge from this brief historical review.

First, we now accept and perhaps take for granted that clinical expertise is prerequisite for most nursing faculty in higher education. We think that nursing practice must be effectively melded with education and research goals. As can be seen from this review of the last 50 years of academic nursing practice, this is a change in self-image and concept for nursing faculty. It was only after a generation's experience with balancing teaching, research, and practice that nurse educators began to fully internalize this changed self-image.

Second, to implement a tripartite mission, schools must find ways to link revenues from teaching, practice, research, and philanthropy to build viable and balanced budgets based on all sources. Until the 1980s, nursing budgets were derived almost entirely from tuition or curriculum-related grants. Ensuring income from research and from reimbursed practice while seeking support from donors for innovations is a relatively recent experience for schools of nursing and continues to pose complex problems of continuity and control.

Third, faculties of the future will continue to maintain their flexibility, recognizing and responding promptly to environmental changes such as new knowledge and technology, gain or loss of revenue streams, and demands for growth or shrinkage regarding their areas of expertise. Consider the impact of the changes in higher education and in nursing practice over the last 30 years. Think of what it meant to individual faculty as curricula changed and relentless demands were made for new clinical skills or research expertise. Readiness to respond when the context changes is fundamental to longevity, but it can be very hard on people.

Looking at the past, then, it would seem that faculties should think of academic nursing practice as both a work in progress and as the best evidence of the rapid development of higher education in nursing over the last 50 years. In so many ways, it is the essence of nursing's high-wire act in today's world. In another decade or so, we will better see how well we accomplished what we set out to do so many decades ago.

REFERENCES

Brown, E. L. (1948). *Nursing for the future: A report prepared for the National Nursing Council*. New York: Russell Sage Foundation.

Clinician educator track in the school of nursing (1984, April 13). *University of Pennsylvania Almanac, 4*(5).

Cohen, A. M. (1998). *The shaping of American higher education: Emergence and growth of the contemporary system*. San Francisco: Jossey-Bass.

Fagin, C. M. (1986). Institutionalizing faculty practice. *Nursing Outlook, 34*(3), 140–144.

Fairman, J., & Lynaugh, J. (1998). *Critical care nursing: A history*. Philadelphia: University of Pennsylvania Press.

Lowery, B. J. (1983, October). *Knowledge builders: Faculty appointments*. Paper presented to Sigma Theta Tau, International, Washington, DC.

Lynaugh, J., & Brush, B. (1996). *American nursing: From hospital to health systems.* Cambridge, MA and Oxford, UK: Blackwell.

University of Pennsylvania School of Nursing & Hospital of the University of Pennsylvania Division of Nursing (April 1984). *Partnership in nursing: For education, practice and Research—A joint proposal.* Philadelphia: University of Pennsylvania School of Nursing and Hospital Division of Nursing.

University of Pennsylvania School of Nursing (April 1997). *1997 Self study.* Philadelphia: Author.

U.S. Surgeon General Consultant Group on Nursing (1963). *Toward quality in nursing.* Washington, DC: U.S. Public Health Service.

Chapter 3

Academic Nursing Practice Models and Related Strategic Issues

Juliann G. Sebastian, Marcia Stanhope, and Carolyn A. Williams

Exemplars by Bonita Ann Pilon, Hila Richardson, and M. Dee Williams

Since their beginnings in the 1960s, academic nursing practices have become a more widespread element of the mission and activities of schools of nursing (Barger, Nugent, & Bridges, 1992). Despite concerns about faculty role strain (Boettcher, 1996) and competition of practice activities with school resources (Lang, Evans, & Swan, 2002), little is known about the strategic impact choices of practice models might have on the other missions of schools. The purpose here is to present a framework for thinking about the structure of academic nursing practice programs and the related strategic impacts. Using a conceptual framework based in organizational and clinical sciences, this chapter examines the relationships between the models developed by schools of nursing for their academic nursing practice programs and the strategic risks and benefits associated with these models. The ideas developed here are part of a larger project that includes a national survey of schools of nursing to be reported subsequently.

Schools of nursing use widely differing models for their practice programs, accruing different risks and benefits from these choices. Even when a school does not make a deliberate choice about academic practice models and instead develops its practices as opportunities arise (Barger, personal communication, April 20, 2002), it is making de facto choices. Mintzberg and Waters (1985) argued that the most relevant organizational strategies emerge over time, rather than from formal strategic planning, and result from individual decisions that together make up a pattern of strategic choices. By contrast, Porter (Argyres & McGahan, 2002) posits that even when strategies emerge, organizational leaders must make choices about strategic directions and conclusions regarding whether individual opportunities fit into an overall strategic direction. Thus, while schools of nursing may not deliberately choose a single practice model, they may construct a portfolio over time containing various models best suited to local opportunities, political realities, and strategic directions of the school.

DEFINITION AND GOALS OF ACADEMIC NURSING PRACTICES

Academic nursing practices can be defined as those practice arrangements that support clinical work "by faculty in schools of nursing and advance the field by consciously and consistently using, facilitating and supporting contemporary research, generating new insights and clinical questions, and developing leaders in the field" (University of Kentucky College of Nursing, 2002a). In a seminal paper presented at an American Academy of Nursing symposium on nursing faculty practice, Ford and Kitzman (1983) stated that "faculty practice refers to those functions performed by faculty within a service setting that have as their principal goal the continued advancement of the nursing care of patients/clients, a goal congruent with the role of an academician in a professional discipline" (p. 14). Such practices promote the development and utilization of new science related to nursing care delivery through the "intentional integration of the tripartite mission of research, education and clinical care in an academic setting" (Lang, Evans, & Swan, 2002, p. 63). From the perspective of individual faculty members, it is practice that is an integral part of a faculty member's work as an academician, rather than an addition to the usual faculty load (Ford & Kitzman, 1985). For example, moonlighting is not considered part of faculty practice according to this definition (Barger, Nugent, & Bridges, 1992). Likewise, academic clinical faculty practice is not simply a byproduct of teaching or research. While academic faculty practice contributes to these goals, the purpose is not limited to any one of them.

Numerous goals for academic nursing practice have been cited in the literature (see, for example, the description of goals by Aydellote and Gregory, 1989). These include providing laboratories for research and development of nursing care delivery innovations (Zachariah & Lundeen, 1997); opportunities for student learning in innovative care delivery sites (Holman & Branstetter, 1997); venues for modeling expert nursing care by faculty for nursing students and interdisciplinary colleagues (Jacobson, MacRobert, Leon, et al., 1998); opportunities for faculty clinical practice, both to maintain currency and to meet requirements for clinical certification; nursing services designed to reduce health disparities by providing care for underserved populations (Boccuzzi, 1998); a source of revenue for the school (McNiel & Mackey, 1995); and improvements in health outcomes for local populations. These goals are not shared by every school, however; those of individual schools likely reflect the school's mission, local opportunities, and availability of funding. If the aims of these programs vary, what then are the underlying conceptual threads that link them? Which considerations are useful for informing a school's decisions about models of practice? How do these considerations vary over time as a school's academic practice initiatives grow, develop and change? An examination follows of the organizational and clinical conceptual bases for models used in academic nursing practices.

CONCEPTUAL BASES OF ACADEMIC NURSING PROGRAMS

Thompson's (1964) seminal work on organizational structure focused attention on relationships between decisions about structure and function and the environmental contexts within which individual organizations are located. He suggested that structural decisions should use a contingency approach, taking into account the unique nature of the context, including the environment, the people and the nature of the work. Such an approach integrates the distinctive combinations of conditions in the environment external to the organization and within the organization itself.

Contingencies are variables that influence an outcome, just as an independent variable influences a dependent variable. In this case the outcome is optimal achievement of the school's academic nursing practice goals. The concept of a contingency is broader than the concept of risk because some contingencies may be opportunities and others may simply be factors that influence the functioning of an aspect of organizational work. The relationships between internal and external organizational contingencies, models of academic nursing practice, and dimensions of the strategic benefits and risks associated with the practice model are highlighted in Figure 3.1.

Contingency theory proposes that there is no single optimal approach for designing organizational structure and functioning. Instead, organizational leaders evaluate a constellation of variables in constructing structures and processes for accomplishing organizational goals. This places heavy demands on the analytic and decision-making abilities of organizational leaders.

Regarding the contingencies facing individual schools of nursing, no single model of academic nursing practice is likely to work best for all schools. Instead, a contingency approach to constructing a model or set of models (a portfolio practice approach) is more likely to lead to optimal outcomes because such an approach accounts for local conditions and unique combinations of needs, constraints, and opportunities. Because a contingency approach considers combinations of variables internal and external to an organization, such an approach offers only limited predictions about the outcomes of specific organizational models. Therefore, decision makers should include analysis of potential strategic benefits and risks likely to accrue as they construct and change their models over time. The emphasis here is on the relationships between the models developed, based on relevant contingencies, and the strategic issues (benefits and risks) that may result.

Relevant Contingencies

Relevant contingencies for academic nursing programs include those originating in the external environment and those from the school's internal environment. Using Thompson's emphases on environment, people, and work, contingencies facing schools of nursing include pressures from the local and national environment, opportunities and needs related to the educational preparation and needs of faculty, and the type of clinical work

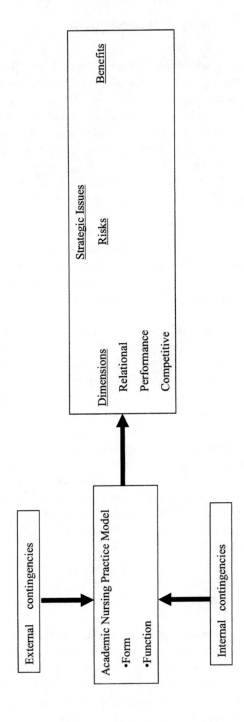

FIGURE 3.1 Relationship between academic nursing practice models and strategic issues.

performed by faculty. For example, environmental factors create regulatory and economic pressures, making reimbursement for advanced practice nursing services more or less risky for schools. Labor market forces may make it difficult to secure adequate funding to cover faculty salaries in practice or, conversely, advanced practice nursing salaries may be so high in a local market that it is difficult to find faculty. Interprofessional issues, such as labor market competition for primary care providers and market pressures from other schools and workplaces, may increase competition for nursing faculty. Finally, the nature of the work is a key contingency, including considerations such as the clinical focus of the work, whether the academic practice model differentiates clinical work across levels of nursing preparation or focuses exclusively on advanced practice, and whether the nursing care is directly reimbursable. For example, a school that operates a population-based program with services differentiated across BSN, MSN, and doctoral levels will most likely need to rely on grants and contracts for funding because such services do not readily lend themselves to fee-for-service reimbursement at this time.

Whether a school is part of a research or a teaching university undoubtedly influences that school's decisions about operating an academic nursing practice, and also its choice among models. Although pressures to allocate resources to research may dampen enthusiasm for academic clinical practice in research intensive universities, the increased access to clinical research opportunities in strong academic clinical programs represents an important consideration. Schools with large advanced practice nursing programs may need the increased access to clinical practice afforded by academic clinical programs for students and faculty alike. If the school of nursing is part of a large university with multiple clinical education programs, other schools within the university may choose to provide clinical services that nursing programs in other universities would be free to pursue. University size and the types of other clinical educational programs present are not the only determinants of which unit offers which clinical services. Political and marketplace pressures likewise enter into such decisions. Examples of programs that may be offered by either nursing or medicine include student or employee health services (Cole & Mackey, 1996), travel clinics (University of Rochester School of Nursing, 2002), or primary care (Boccuzzi, 1998; Spitzer, 1997). Local workforce needs represent an important contingency in decisions about clinical practice opportunities for academic nursing. For example, schools with nurse practitioner or midwifery programs need access to adequate clinical practice opportunities for faculty teaching in these programs, both to ensure ongoing clinical competency and certification and to provide students with appropriate learning laboratories.

Importance of Models for Academic Nursing Practice

Organizational theorists have focused attention on structural arrangements, asking whether these choices determine the way an organization functions, how effectively an organization functions, or whether function should determine form (see, for example, Thompson, 1967). The concept of a model integrates both form and function. A model is a representation of how something works, including what it looks like (structure) and how it operates (function). For example, a business model reflects choices about ownership, financing, clientele, and the way a product or service is made available to clients. Business models include five elements: structure (design), function (how a product or service is delivered), type of product or service, who pays for the product or service, and identification of customers or clients. Similarly, a conceptual model includes decisions about which elements should be included in the model, in what ways these elements are arranged (structure), and how the elements operate together (function) (Dickoff & James, 1968).

Models are important because they represent design choices with significant strategic implications. The choice a school makes about a model for academic nursing practice lays the foundation for the types of risks and benefits the school will face and thereby influences the school's ability to meet its strategic goals. Even when choices are emergent rather than deliberate (Mintzberg & Waters, 1985), and patterns become clear only in retrospect, they still have strategic implications as Porter observes (Argyres & McGahan, 2002). What can schools use to guide choices about a model for academic nursing practice? What types of models have been reported in the literature?

ACADEMIC PRACTICE MODELS

Practice models can be conceptualized based on sites of practice (schools, homes, inpatient care) or form of nursing-care delivery (case management) (Sawyer, Alexander, Gordon, Juszczak, & Gillis, 2000). What has not yet been addressed in the literature is (a) how structure, function, and clientele combine to create a multidimensional model of practice, or (b) the corresponding research questions about how those models influence strategic risks and benefits for the school.

The conceptual dimensions that will be used to evaluate models of nursing practice are (1) the ownership of the practice and its relationship with the parent organization (structure), (2) the measures of performance that are used (function), and (3) the ways in which clientele of the practices are defined (clientele).

Continuum of Ownership

Ownership refers to the extent to which the school of nursing has financial responsibility for, administers, and manages its own practices. Ownership may not reside solely with the school or department but may be shared with a larger organizational enterprise made up of the entire college or university. It may be shared with an outside organization as in a partnership arrangement, or it may be solely owned by another entity. Having responsibility for a practice gives the school of nursing the opportunity to demonstrate unique models of care and to design the conditions under which the practice functions (Lang, Evans, & Swan, 2002). In essence, it allows for *efficacy testing*, or testing innovative nursing-care delivery models in a situation in which the school can control as many variables as possible. Ownership, however, brings with it corresponding responsibilities for infrastructure including staffing responsibilities, legal accountability for the practice as a whole, and financial responsibilities to ensure not only a breakeven position but to generate more revenues than expenses in order to make ongoing improvements to the practice. Ownership or responsibility for the financial, administrative, and managerial aspects of a practice gives the school a form of modified equity in the practice. The practice generates both tangible and intangible benefits for the school but also carries responsibility for the risks.

Contracting with other organizations for faculty members' clinical time is at the other end of the continuum of ownership possibilities. This provides some level of financial security because the other organization provides the infrastructure and overhead for the practice and may do the billing for the faculty member. It may, however, reduce the school's opportunities for generating revenues in excess of expenses if the contract simply covers the school's cost of doing business. Capturing the full cost of providing service by including the overhead associated with administration of the faculty practice averts this problem (Starck, Walker, & Bohannon, 1991), while schools that build a risk-sharing arrangement can generate revenues in addition to expenses that can be used for future innovations. From a clinical perspective, such practice arrangements provide opportunities for *effectiveness testing*, or testing clinical practice models under conditions in which the school of nursing has less control over the clinical environment. These arrangements also may provide for interdisciplinary collaboration and may include collaboration with people or groups outside the health professions, such as teachers, business leaders, or community groups.

The range of ownership possibilities available to a school of nursing can be conceptualized as a continuum, from full equity ownership of a practice (or full financial responsibility for administering and operating the practice) to contractual arrangements wherein other parties own the practice and contract with the school of nursing for faculty service. Between the two ends of the continuum are the unification model, in which faculty have joint responsibilities both to the school of nursing and to the clinical service setting owned by the university (Ford & Kitzman, 1983) and joint clinical appointments (Broussard, Delahoussaye, & Poirrier, 1996). In joint clinical appointments, the parent organization, another department or school, or an affiliating agency owns the practice sites, and nursing faculty hold joint clinical appointments with those other units. An example of such appointments is the case when nursing faculty hold joint clinical faculty appointments in the medical school.

Performance Measures

The primary performance measures used by a practice are likely to play a prominent role in how the practice functions, because performance measures create visibility and incentives. Measures of effectiveness provide some indication of the key values held by an organization (Yuchtman & Seashore, 1967) and suggest how the organization will function to achieve those particular indicators. Organizational effectiveness in health care may be measured using output, outcome, or some combination of the two types of measures (Omachanu, 1989). Outputs are units of service delivery, such as volume indicators. Numbers of individual clients seen, numbers of visits or hospitalizations, and numbers of programs are all indicators of outputs. Outcomes reflect changes in health status and may be measured using the defined clientele as the unit of analysis. For example, changes in individual health status as a result of interventions (Donabedian, 1988); changes in family, group, or community-level health status; or changes in population health status as measured by incidence and prevalence rates may all be measures of outcomes using a range of levels of analysis. In most practice models, a combination of outputs and outcomes is likely to be used, placing the school's practices somewhere along the continuum rather than distinctly at one end or the other. For example, Mackey & McNiel (2002) recommend a comprehensive set of quality indicators for academic nursing centers (in particular) that include a heavy focus on the structure and processes of care. They suggest a range of indicators, including the nature of clinical, administrative, and educational policies and procedures, as well as indicators of client and staff satisfaction. Their recommendations would place a nursing center closer to the midpoint of the output-outcome dimension of performance measures.

Clientele

The way a school defines its clientele influences the model of practice. Clients may be defined in terms of the unit of analysis, from individuals to families, groups, communities, and populations. For example, a school of nursing might operate a primary care clinic and provide services to individuals, maintaining individual client charts and accounting for volume in part by the number of individuals served (Sawyer, Alexander, Gordon, et al., 2000). This type of arrangement creates the opportunity to bill public and commercial payers for services, but carries with it corresponding legal obligations regarding structural arrangements and exposes the school to greater risks. Likewise, a portfolio might include a family-focused nursing center with family charts, a health education and screening practice aimed at groups such as employees in an occupational setting, and/or a community (such as a neighborhood), or a population-focused practice in which populations may be defined based on age (e.g., children or older adults), gender (women's health), health problem (e.g., heart failure), or cultural or linguistic patterns (e.g., Spanish speaking). Choices the school makes about clientele contribute to decisions about practice ownership and performance practice measures. For example, a population-focused practice may emphasize population level outcomes rather than outputs (such as number of unduplicated clients served) owing to the difficulty collecting data on these indicators. The dimension underlying the clientele continuum is not the numbers of people included in a single category but the degree of abstraction in the category. For example, a community might contain more people than a population, but because a community may have more definitive boundaries (particularly if defined geographically), a population has a higher level of abstraction.

STRATEGIC ISSUES ASSOCIATED WITH MODELS OF ACADEMIC NURSING PRACTICE

Strategic issues (i.e., potential risks and benefits) associated with models of academic nursing practice are analyzed along three dimensions (Das & Sheng-Teng, 1999): relational, performance, and competitive position. These dimensions are illustrated in Figure 1 as part of the relationship between academic nursing practice models and strategic issues. The relational dimension is concerned with issues originating from the extent of commitment by various participants in the activity and the dynamics that emerge when working with organizational partners. The performance dimension refers to both financial and clinical performance and addresses issues of risk and quality. Competitive advantage explains a school of nursing's ability to take advantage of opportunities when they are available and to use those opportunities to most fully meet the mission of the school.

Relational Benefits and Risks

To achieve their missions, schools of nursing are increasingly looking toward partnerships that include relevant constituencies in designing programs and making decisions (Barger, 1999; Sebastian & Chappell, 1998). Benefits of partnerships can include decision making that is more creative or more inclusive because diverse perspectives have been considered (Gale, 1998). Partnerships can yield support that had not previously existed from organizations and coalitions. Partnerships have their own dynamics, however, and may result in dyads, triads, or even larger sets of linkages in which partners hold asymmetrical levels of commitment to the clinical ventures. Likewise, partnerships require significant amounts of time and energy to encourage shared definitions of problems and needs, to include relevant input into decision making, and to maintain effective communication over time (Sebastian, Skelton, & West, 2000; see also Chapters 11 & 12).

Performance Benefits and Risks

Performance benefits and risks associated with varying academic nursing practice models center on concerns related to clinical quality and financial risk. In situations in which high levels of clinical quality can be documented through clinical information systems and well-designed evaluation plans, schools of nursing can succeed in developing effective new care delivery models and provide students and researchers with unique learning laboratories. The contributions to local communities and improved health status in such situations are noteworthy (Naylor & Buhler-Wilkerson, 1999), as is the ability to influence health services and policy at state and federal levels. Administering one's own practice makes it easier to control the conditions for practice and presumably to control the levels of quality. Ownership, however, requires a solid infrastructure (see Chapter 7). Ownership also requires access to sufficient capital through grants or loans to build the practice to the breakeven point and to buffer it in situations in which cash flow is reduced. Without such a cushion, clinical quality could be reduced.

On the other hand, while contracting with other agencies for faculty practice opportunities reduces some of these demands, contracting also places the school of nursing at arm's length from full control over model building, quality improvement, and policy making. Another consideration is that other agencies may have staffing and scheduling needs that conflict with the school's need for the faculty member to participate in teaching and research programs or in school or professional service commitments.

Financial risk and accountability is greatest when schools own their own practices, although in some cases the potential financial benefit may also be greatest when the school assumes this risk. Ownership of a practice provides the opportunity to retain billable revenues in excess of expenses. The expenses and financial accountability associated with such an approach, however, are greater than when contracting with other agencies. Schools with multiple models of practice or a practice portfolio approach may be able to diversify their financial risks. For example, owning a practice and assuming responsibility for generating adequate revenues to both operate and improve the practice over time places a substantial financial burden on a school. Changes in the regulatory or political environment may influence a practice's viability. Evans and Yurkow (1999) describe the impact that the Balanced Budget Act (BBA) of 1997 had on The CARE Program for frail elders operated by the University of Pennsylvania School of Nursing.

Changes in reimbursement regulations for Comprehensive Outpatient Rehabilitation Facilities (CORF) that were included in BBA 1997 resulted in closure of this practice.

Competitive Position

A school's competitive orientation and position in the local health care market can influence its choice of a model or models and, likewise, the school's choices may influence its competitive position. Miles and Snow's (1978) typology of organizations' strategic orientations helps explain organizations' competitive positions. They argued that organizations might be characterized by their overall orientations along two dimensions, that is, tendencies toward action and tendencies toward analysis. Organizations with strong propensities toward both action and analysis reflect what Miles and Snow referred to as "prospector" organizations. Those with strong propensities toward action but little orientation toward analysis may be thought of as "defenders," whereas those with little focus on either action or analysis are "reactors." Finally, organizations that emphasize analysis over action may be characterized as "analyzers." While none of the four types is necessarily more likely to lead to organizational success, environmental forces are thought to influence which type is most desirable under a given set of circumstances.

Functioning as a reactor does not favorably position an organization in a dynamic market in which fast and flexible responsiveness is needed. Some schools of nursing that are part of very large institutions may find it difficult to respond rapidly to market shifts, and, furthermore, may value more deliberate and thoughtful responses to market pressures. For example, when a particular model is being evaluated, the school may hesitate to make changes until all the data are collected. Schools that are part of smaller institutions with a strong emphasis on meeting local market needs may find it easier to respond quickly to market demands. Thus, environmental contingencies influence the patterns that emerge within a school's usual manner of functioning.

Similarly, a school's choice of model has the potential to influence its position in the local marketplace. A school with numerous contractual practices is partnering with a wide range of other organizations that may help build interorganizational relationships over time. A school with extensive clinical appointments may be better positioned within its own clinical enterprise to demonstrate decision-making power equal to that of other disciplines and to be a viable collaborator in the context of clinical care. These are important lessons for students and critical observations for those who might be considering nursing as a potential career choice.

Finally, academic clinical practice programs may provide a sort of competitive edge for a school of nursing because, when successful, these programs can increase student access to innovative practice environments, provide opportunities for developing and testing evidence-based practice, and expand access to clinical research opportunities. Thus, the potential exists for academic clinical practice programs to contribute to a school's overall environment of clinical scholarship. Local market conditions, regulatory considerations, and political issues, however, may create sufficiently high entry barriers to dissuade investment in academic clinical nursing practice.

Practice Portfolio Approach

Figure 3.2 depicts a three-dimensional view of the conceptual bases for academic nursing practice models and a sample array of models that might be in place in a school of nursing. Some schools may opt for a single model, while others may develop multiple models as shown. Use of multiple models would constitute a practice portfolio approach to an academic nursing practice.

In the conceptual diagram, a school's practices could be plotted in a three-dimensional space bounded by ownership, performance measures, and clientele. The example reflects a primary care center in which a nursing faculty practice that is owned by another entity has a strong focus on outputs (such as productivity indicators like patient volume or total encounters) as measures of performance and a focus on caring for individuals. The community health center has a stronger emphasis on performance measures of changes in health status; this center includes care for families as well as individuals. Finally, the nursing center depicted is owned and operated by the school of nursing, provides population-focused services, and emphasizes heavily the outputs of nursing care delivery. Each of these scenarios is hypothetical and, taken together, the scenarios illustrate a method for diagramming a set of models in three-dimensional space. A national study is in process that tests the utility of the model proposed here.

Using contingency logic, the questions for schools of nursing relate to the predictive value of examining the effectiveness of a school's practice model or models along these three dimensions in light of the local environ-

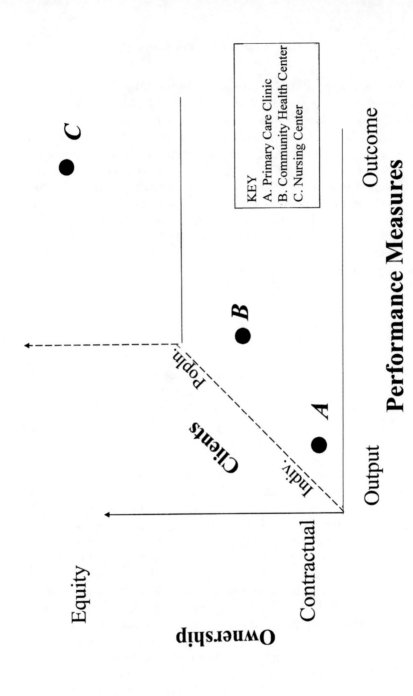

FIGURE 3.2   Conceptual bases of academic nursing practices: Sample portfolio configuration.

KEY
A. Primary Care Clinic
B. Community Health Center
C. Nursing Center

Performance Measures

Output   Outcome

Ownership

Contractual

Equity

Clients

Popln.

Indiv.

52

ment, the faculty and staff working in the practices, and the nature of the work. In the future, therefore, the following research questions may provide answers useful in guiding strategic design choices by schools of nursing:

1. How is academic nursing practice effectiveness influenced by environmental factors?
2. How is fiscal viability related to the practice portfolio configuration and local economic and regulatory conditions?
3. Which models support evidence-based practice and ongoing clinical improvements by academic nursing and under what circumstances?
4. Which models best facilitate achievement of the educational, clinical, and research goals of academic nursing?
5. Which practice models yield the best outcomes to key societal concerns (e.g., reduction of health disparities, attracting students to nursing, stimulating students' use of evidence in practice, and enhancing quality in care delivery)?
6. How do academic nursing practices change throughout various stages of development?

Examination of several different practices highlight issues analyzed in this chapter. The practice at the University of Kentucky College of Nursing is examined in depth. Practices from three additional schools (Vanderbilt University, New York University, and University of Florida) will exemplify these themes (see Exemplars A, B, and C).

UNIVERSITY OF KENTUCKY COLLEGE OF NURSING ACADEMIC NURSING PRACTICE

History

The University of Kentucky College of Nursing Academic Nursing Practice formally originated in 1984 when Carolyn A. Williams joined the college as dean. One of her goals was to stimulate the growth of a viable faculty practice program that would contribute to the teaching, research, and service missions of the school. From the beginning, the college aimed to develop a diverse portfolio of practice initiatives. College practice activities filled niches not assumed by others in the health care arena. Essentially, the college chose to seize opportunities as they became available and match those opportunities with faculty who would find them rewarding and highly consistent with their clinical expertise and scholarly interests. The strategy was one of developing a series of successes and maximizing opportunities. Practice activities started modestly and with limited, albeit real, capital investments when the practice opportunities advanced college goals.

The first organized, revenue-generating practice was a nurse-managed clinic for homeless adults that had been initiated as a volunteer student project in 1981 by Eva Smith, then an RN-BSN student in the College of Nursing. In 1985, the college began operating the clinic with funding from the board of the Community Kitchen, a nonprofit organization that provided services for the homeless population. This was followed by a Federal Division of Nursing Special Projects Grant awarded to Marcia Stanhope (1986–1989). The College of Nursing faculty ran the clinic and provided learning experiences for BSN and MSN students and research opportunities for doctoral students and faculty.

Numerous other practice activities were developed throughout the ensuing years, including contracts for nursing services and other nurse-led services operated by the College of Nursing, such as a parish nursing program in a local faith community (Berry, 2000) and a nursing care management program for families with medically fragile children. A wide range of collaborative relationships developed over time, including an early nursing administration and research faculty role with a geriatric home-visiting program that was part of the university's Sanders-Brown Center on Aging; pediatric nurse practitioner staffing for a comprehensive family care center providing educational and health services for low income families; and family nurse practitioner services with the university's Department of Family Practice, numerous private physician practices, and several health departments. In some cases, particular practices were phased out either because the practice was mature and ready to be institutionalized within another organization or because the necessary faculty expertise was no longer available. As each practice developed, students were involved, and open discussions occurred among faculty so that all could learn the organizational, clinical, and economic details that influence the viability of nursing services.

By 1994, faculty in the College of Nursing voted to approve a formal faculty practice plan (University of Kentucky Administrative Regulations, 1994). This legal instrument defines membership in the plan, clinical practice rights and responsibilities of plan participants, and management of revenues and protection of financial solvency. In 1996, the dean appointed an assistant dean for advanced practice, Juliann Sebastian, whose responsibilities include the college's academic nursing practice program.

In 1999, Dr. Sebastian, two faculty members, and the college's director of business affairs, Karen Minton, were awarded Penn-Macy fellowships to participate in the further development of the concept of academic nursing practice.

A key event that stimulated new ideas and development of innovative forms of practice occurred in 1998 when the college's associate dean, Marcia Stanhope, received a grant from a local philanthropy, the Good Samaritan Foundation, to establish an integrated nursing center. The center was named the Good Samaritan Nursing Center for Health Promotion and Illness Prevention in honor of the foundation that has provided continuous grant funding since that time. The center brings together the work of community health nursing interns and nurse practitioner fellows along with faculty and staff from the College of Nursing. Center staff members provide professional and advanced practice nursing care in 11 community-based settings for the purpose of improving the health of underserved local populations (Stanhope, 2001). These settings include nurse-managed school-based and community clinics, neighborhood and free clinics, and one countywide health promotion project.

Current Status

Practice portfolio model. The College of Nursing continues to use numerous approaches to academic nursing practice, reflecting opportunities, philosophy, and capacities. Roughly 60% of the college's practice revenues come from grants and contracts supporting the college owned and operated Good Samaritan Nursing Center for Health Promotion and Illness Prevention. Another 15% comes from contracts with external agencies, and approximately 25% from clinical appointments within the medical center. This portfolio allows the college to spread the risks associated with clinical practice, while providing opportunities for efficacy and effectiveness testing of nursing care delivery models in both intra- and interdisciplinary environments.

Strategic issues. Strategic issues for the college's Academic Clinical Program relate to fulfillment of the college's tripartite mission for education, research, and service. Using Das and Sheng-Teng's (1999) categorization of strategic issues related to alliances, the practice portfolio of the college may be analyzed in terms of relational, performance, and competitive positional risks and benefits.

From the perspective of relational risks and benefits, the college is interconnected with a wide range of other organizations with every clinical initiative in which it is engaged, including those related to the college-owned-and-operated Good Samaritan Nursing Center. Risks related to achieving the college's mission include finding ways to advance the missions of both the college and the partner agency, managing smooth communication flow across agencies, and developing and refining policies that reflect the needs, legal issues, and concerns of partner agencies. On the other hand, benefits are numerous and include expanding access to clinical sites for learning and research, maintaining high levels of awareness of and involvement with contemporary clinical trends, and participating in an active and ongoing way in improvement of local health-related quality of life.

In terms of performance risks, the college has more degrees of freedom over the Good Samaritan Nursing Center than over the contractual relationships and the clinical appointments. This allows for more opportunities to design and test new approaches to care delivery. It also places the responsibility for policies related to personnel, clinical services, and administrative matters with the college. A key performance asset is that the college has numerous opportunities for clinical scholarship from its many practice activities. One issue is the development of formalized mechanisms for ongoing evaluation of each practice initiative separately and all components of the Academic Clinical Program jointly. Because so many different organizational entities relate to the college, it is often challenging to develop programwide approaches for continuous clinical improvement. Despite the need to customize evaluation and clinical improvements somewhat to the different practice settings, a major performance benefit is the opportunity this broad practice base provides for research in arrangements that, in the aggregate, function much like a practice-based research network (Deshefy-Longhi, Swartz, & Grey, 2002; see also Chapters 9 & 12).

Finally, its highly diversified academic clinical program places the college in a more stable and advantageous competitive position than if it relied on one model of practice alone. Having used this strategy since the beginning created a strong foundation for the college's expansion of its practice activities. The many diverse practice initiatives provide educational and research opportunities for students that both enrich students' learning experiences and provide avenues for student recruitment. Efforts are underway to develop new strategies for expanding educational opportunities to ensure that students in each of the college's programs from the BSN through the two doctoral programs (PhD and Doctor of Nursing Practice) will have learning experiences in one or more of its practices. By 2001–2002, over 50% of the college's nurse practitioner students had at least one learning experience in a college faculty practice setting, compared with 24% in 1999–2000 (U.K. College of Nursing, 2002b). In spring 2001, the college began offering practicum experiences in its practices to high-school students who expressed interest in nursing and were enrolled in the countywide Experience-Based Career Education Program. The aim of this initiative is to interest students in both undergraduate and graduate education and subsequent career opportunities. Two of these students were admitted the college's BSN program in 2002.

Given its propensity both for action (developing new practice opportunities on a regular basis) and analysis (evaluating outcomes of practice activities), the college's strategic orientation tends toward Miles and Snow's Prospector Typology; there is always, however, a necessary balance between a penchant for action and for analysis. In publicly funded land-grant institutions such as the University of Kentucky, the mission supports outreach and development of diverse learning experiences such as those available with the college's academic clinical program. The college is part of a strong research-intensive environment, with its classification as a Carnegie Research I institution and Kentucky's mandate to the university to expand its research programs (Kentucky Higher Education Reform Act, 1997). This environment promotes an emphasis on analysis, critique and dissemination of evaluation and research emanating from the clinical practices.

Other Examples

Three additional schools of nursing have shared synopses of their academic clinical programs and the strategic issues arising from the models they have chosen for their practices. These are Vanderbilt University School of Nursing, New York University Division of Nursing, and the University of Florida College of Nursing—exemplars A, B, and C, respectively. Each exemplar highlights unique strengths and local pressures that influenced the schools' choice of practice models and the attendant strategic issues.

CONCLUSION

While more needs to be known about the nature and types of relationships between the conceptual models on which schools of nursing base their practices, the ensuing strategic risks and benefits, and the changes in these configurations over time, case descriptions of several programs suggest that strategic issues do relate to the models schools develop and that these issues are likewise related to the context in which the school is functioning. Strategic issues can yield benefits for schools of nursing but carry with them certain costs or risks that must be addressed and managed. Research is needed to further develop and validate the conceptual framework proposed in this chapter and to clarify the extent and nature of the benefits and costs of the models schools choose under differing local political, economic, and cultural circumstances.

Acknowledgments

Portions of this work were made possible in part through support from the Robert Wood Johnson Nurse Executive Fellowship Program to the first author (J. Sebastian) and the Good Samaritan Foundation, Inc., to the second author (M. Stanhope). The authors gratefully acknowledge the suggestions made by Fellows of the Penn-Macy Initiative to Advance Academic Nursing Practice and participants in the American Association of Colleges of Nursing Faculty Practice Conference, February 23, 2001. Appreciation is extended to Sue Pope and Said Abu-Salem, research assistants to Dr. Sebastian, who helped with various stages of this project.

Exemplar A.
Use of a Practice Portfolio Approach for Faculty Practice at Vanderbilt University School of Nursing.

Vanderbilt University School of Nursing (VUSN) uses the Practice Portfolio Approach delineated in this Chapter to describe and analyze its practice program. Currently, VUSN operates nurse-managed centers at nine sites in metropolitan Nashville. In addition, VUSN runs a full-scope midwifery service with deliveries at Vanderbilt University Hospital. Various individual contract practices exist within and outside the medical center.

Each practice can be easily classified as equity, contract, and/or grant. Over the past two years there has been a strategic shift toward combining funding sources rather than relying on a single source of capital. Equity models represent the greatest financial risk to VUSN. Revenue is dependent on the local reimbursement market for nurse practitioners and nurse midwives as well as on patient volume. Credentialing and billing infrastructures must be in place and highly efficient. Lines of credit are required in order to maintain solvency during some months. At VUSN, financial backup is provided by the school with approval of the university. For FY 2003, practice expenses in the equity model are projected at $1.6M for the nurse-managed centers and $470,000 for the nurse midwifery practice. Profits or losses are posted in the VUSN financial report.

Some practices are solely grant funded and many combine grant funding and equity. The latter are practices that receive Division of Nursing training funds and are also billing for services delivered. School health clinics typify this type of practice model. Practices that are 100% grant funded pose no financial risk; long-term sustainability, however, is almost always a challenge.

Contract practices are the most stable model and generally show a small profit. VUSN routinely contracts with outside agencies and community physician practices for faculty practice time. Within Vanderbilt Medical Center, the school of nursing uses memoranda of understanding to place faculty nurse practitioners in collaborative practice arrangements in the medical center clinics and hospital. These internal arrangements are for salary and benefits only. Any revenue generated by the nurse faculty member is kept by the agency or clinic that contracts with VUSN.

Thus, the portfolio at Vanderbilt University School of Nursing contains a number of different practices and is more complex than that at schools with single models. This portfolio would more closely resemble the diagram in Figure 3.2, with its multiple practices and differing ownership, performance measures, and client bases, than would a school with a single practice model.

—Bonnie Pilon

Exemplar B.
The NYU Division of Nursing Academic Nursing Practice Model.

In 1998, the Division of Nursing in New York University's Steinhardt School of Education initiated a contractual model of academic nursing practice. Using this model, the division has maintained from 8 to 15 contracts with community-based agencies and health providers since the beginning of the program. The model combines full- or part-time clinical faculty practice in the agencies, referred to as community partners, with clinical instruction of graduate and undergraduate nursing students. The contracts cover the cost of the salary and fringe benefits for the faculty member plus an administrative fee that ranges from 3% to 5% of the contract costs.

This model was selected because it offered the opportunity to develop a variety of community-based opportunities for innovative nurse practitioner roles. For example, some of the contracts are for psychiatric nurse practitioners working with adult populations in mental health clinics or continuing day treatment, some are for pediatric nurse practitioners in comprehensive school-based clinics, and some are for family nurse practitioners in agencies serving homeless or other vulnerable populations. Another important reason for this particular model is that it poses minimal financial risk to the division. The amount of funding specified in the contracts cover the total proportional costs for salary and fringe benefits for the faculty member. The division does not have to cover any operational costs and is at minimal risk for regulatory requirements at the sites. Further, the model does not require any capital from the division or the university to develop the practices. The only cost to the division is the salary of the director who manages the program.

The model has many advantages. It offers access to a variety of innovative practice roles and settings for students, depending on their future practice interests, and it provides faculty with a combined role in innovative practice and teaching. The model provides an opportunity to improve nursing practice and expand health care services in community agencies, and it increases the division's visibility in the community through the partnerships. It offers access to population-based research opportunities, is self-funded, offers community agencies and health care providers an option to introduce new services at lower risk because of outsourcing, and provides community-based agencies with a higher quality nurse practitioner than might be possible without the academic linkage available through this model.

Implementation and management of the model has not been without challenges and issues. Among them has been the difficulty in some cases of integrating a nurse practitioner role in agencies that are not health care providers and that use other than medical models of practice. Also, the lack of direct administrative and clinical oversight in the agency has *prevented monitoring of practice quality, the changing of policies and procedures, or the introducing of research. Finally, a significant amount of management time is often required to make such an entrepreneurial model fit into an academic administrative structure more accustomed to grant rather than contract funding approaches. The model has been very successful for the division, for its students and faculty, and for the community agencies involved. The benefits continue to far outweigh the risks and challenges. This model lies on the contractual end of the ownership continuum—toward the left side of the performance measures axis and toward the front of the clientele axis in the conceptual diagram in Figure 3.2.*

—Hila Richardson

Exemplar C.
The University of Florida Shands Eastside
Community Practice.

The University of Florida Shands Eastside Community Practice (ECP) was established in 1997 with the goal of providing interdisciplinary community-based primary health care and health professions education. Located in northeast Gainesville about four miles from the University of Florida Health Science Center, the ECP building was renovated by Shands HealthCare and later donated to the university. Consisting of approximately 11,000 square feet, the building is divided into a family and pediatric practice section and a dental practice section with common waiting room, reception area, medical records area, staff lounge, and administrative offices.

The professional provider team includes faculty members from the colleges of nursing, dentistry, pharmacy, health professions, and medicine. Students from each of these disciplines complete clinical rotations under faculty supervision. Clinical and clerical support services are provided via contract with Shands HealthCare. Clinical services include family and pediatric primary care, pediatric and adult dental care, social work, clinical pharmacy, clinical and health psychology, and psychiatric–mental health nursing. A director of educational and community programs organizes health education sessions and health fairs throughout the East Gainesville community to promote preventive health care and provide support groups for persons with chronic illnesses. Faculty members from the ECP are often speakers at these health forums.

Governance and budget for the ECP are the responsibility of the University of Florida vice president for health affairs. Revenue from a variety of sources supports the practice. An annual appropriation from the Florida legislature, patient revenue, AHEC funds, a contribution from Shands HealthCare, Department of Health funds, corporate donations, and cash or in-kind contributions from each of the five colleges also support the ECP. The Eastside Oversight Committee, consisting of representatives from each of the five participating colleges, Shands HealthCare, AHEC, and the east Gainesville community at-large, serves as the policy-making body for the ECP.

The ECP patient population is diverse and challenging. Dental patients are primarily children with Medicaid coverage. Family practice patients are predominately adults, some of whom require only preventive and episodic care and others of whom require the management of multiple, chronic illnesses. Approximately 50% of these patients have Medicare and/or Medicaid health care coverage, 25% have other third-party payers, 15% are unable to pay, and the remaining 10% are self-pay. Pediatric patients are primarily covered by Medicaid; a few have health care coverage with other third party payers. Over 10,000 patient visits with ECP's family and pediatric interdisciplinary providers are projected for FY 2002–2003.

ECP lies approximately halfway on the contractual-equity continuum on the practice portfolio model (See Fig. 3.2). No single entity "owns" the practice; rather, there are multiple stakeholders with letters of agreement and one formal contract that describe their relationships to ECP. Stakeholders include five health science center deans and department chairs, Shands HealthCare, AHEC, the Florida legislature, east Gainesville residents, and the provider-staff team.

When established, ECP had several goals. These included interdisciplinary team practice; high quality, cost-effective primary care, disease prevention and health promotion, decreased nonurgent use of area emergency departments, services for paying and nonpaying patients, and interdisciplinary health professions education.

The practice lies about midway on the outputs-outcomes continuum (see Fig. 3.2) as well. Measurable outputs include provider productivity goals, dollar value of unfunded care, number of participating health professions students, and number of emergency department patients re-

ferred to ECP. The groundwork has been laid for measurement of the following outcomes:

- *Impact on the general health status of the east Gainesville community,*
- *Tracking increases or decreases in nonurgent emergency department visits by ECP patients,*
- *Effectiveness of interdisciplinary care in the treatment of patients with chronic diseases.*

Barriers to the measurement of outcomes include lack of funds to support another in-depth follow-up community health assessment, lack of staff and of compatible information systems to track emergency department utilization patterns, and limited faculty time to evaluate the interdisciplinary model of care.

Finally, with its emphasis on individual clients but some population-focused health education and screening activities, it is roughly in the middle of the clientele axis (Fig. 3.2). While this is a single model practice and more easily represented on the conceptual model than is a portfolio practice approach, the complexity originates in the number of partners involved in the practice, the range of services, and the mix in types of clientele (individuals and groups).

—M. Dee Williams

REFERENCES

Argyres, N., & McGahan, A. M. (2002). An interview with Michael Porter. *Academy of Management Executive, 16*(2), 43–52.

Aydellote, M., & Gregory, M. (1989). Nursing practice: Innovative models. In *Nursing centers: Meeting the demand for quality health care* (Publication no. 21-2311). New York: National League for Nursing.

Barger, S. E., Nugent, K. E., & Bridges, W. C. (1992). Nursing faculty practice: An organizational perspective. *Journal of Professional Nursing, 8*(5), 263–270.

Barger, S. E. (1999). Partnerships for practice: A necessity in the new millennium. *Journal of Professional Nursing, 15*(4), 208.

Berry, R. (2000). Community health nurses as parish nurses and block nurses. In M. Stanhope & J. Lancaster, *Community health nursing: Process and practice for promoting health* (5th ed.). St. Louis: C. V. Mosby.

Boccuzzi, N. K. (1998). CAPNA: A new development to increase quality in primary care. *Nursing Administration Quarterly, 22*(4), 11–19.

Boettcher, J. H. (1996). Nurse practice centers in academia: An emerging subsystem. *Journal of Nursing Education, 35*(2), 63–68.

Broussard, A. B., Delahoussaye, C. P., & Poirrier, G. P. (1996). The practice role in the academic nursing community. *Journal of Nursing Education, 35*(2), 82–87.

Cole, F. L., & Mackey, T. (1996). Utilization of an academic nursing center. *Journal of Professional Nursing, 12*(6), 349–353.

Das, T. K., & Sheng Teng, B. (1999). Managing risks in strategic alliances. *The Academy of Management Executive, 13*(4), 50–60.

Deshefy-Longhi, T., Swartz, M. K., & Grey, M. (2002). Establishing a practice-based research network of advanced practice registered nurses in southern New England. *Nursing Outlook, 50*(3), 127–132.

Dickoff, J., & James, P. (1968). Symposium on theory development in nursing. A theory of theories: A position paper. *Nursing Research, 17*(3), 197–203.

Donabedian, A. (1988). The quality of care. How can it be assessed? *Journal of the American Medical Association, 260*(12), 1743–1748.

Evans, L. K., & Yurkow, J. (1999). Balanced budget act of 1997 impact on a nurse-managed academic nursing practice for frail elders. *Nursing Economic$, 17*(5), 279–282.

Ford, L. C., & Kitzman, H. J. (1983). Organizational perspectives on faculty practice: Issues and challenges. *The first annual symposium on nursing faculty practice: Structure to outcome, Making it work.* Kansas City, MO: American Academy of Nursing.

Gale, B. J. (1998). Faculty practice as partnership with a community coalition. *Journal of Professional Nursing, 14*(5), 267–271.

Holman, E. J., & Branstetter, E. (1997). An academic nursing center's financial survival. *Nursing Economic$, 15*(5), 248–252.

Jacobson, S. F., MacRobert, M., Leon, C., & McKennon, E. (1998). A faculty case management practice: Integrating teaching, service and research. *Nursing and Health Care Perspectives, 19*(5), 220–223.

Kentucky Higher Education Reform Act. (1997).

Lang, N. M., Evans, L. K., & Swan, B. A. (2002). Penn Macy initiative to advance academic nursing practice. *Journal of Professional Nursing, 18,* 63–69.

McNiel, N. O., & Mackey, T. A. (1995). The consistency of change in the development of nursing faculty practice plans. *Journal of Professional Nursing, 11*(4), 220–226.

Mackey, T. A., & McNiel, N. O. (2002). Quality indicators for academic nursing primary care centers. *Nursing Economic$, 20*(2), 62–65, 73.

Miles, R. E., & Snow, C. C. (1978). *Organizational strategy, structure and process.* New York: McGraw-Hill.

Mintzberg, H., & Waters, J. (1985). Of strategies, deliberate and emergent. *Strategic Management Journal, 6,* 257–262.

Naylor, M. D., & Buhler-Wilkerson, K. (1999). Creating community-based care for the new millennium. *Nursing Outlook, 47*(3), 120–127.

Omachonu, V. K., & Nanda, R. (1989). Measuring productivity: Outcome vs. output. *Nursing Management, 20*(4), 35–40.

Sawyer, M., Alexander, I., Gordon, L., Juszczak, L., & Gilliss, C. (2000). A critical review of current nursing faculty practice. *Journal of the American Academy of Nurse Practitioners, 12*(12), 511–516.

Sebastian, J. G., Davis, R. R., & Chappell, H. (1998). Academia as partner in organizational change. *Nursing Administration Quarterly, 23*(1), 62–71.

Sebastian, J. G., Skelton, J., & West, K. P. (2000). Principle 7: There is feedback to, among and from all stakeholders in the partnership, with the goal of continuously improving the partnership and its outcomes. *Partnership Perspectives, 1*(11), 57–64.

Spitzer, R. (1997). The Vanderbilt University experience. *Nursing Management, 28*(3), 38–40.

Stanhope, M. (2001). *Annual report. University of Kentucky College of Nursing Good Samaritan Nursing Center for Health Promotion and Illness Prevention.* Lexington, KY: University of Kentucky College of Nursing.

Starck, P. L., Walker, G. C., & Bohannon, P. A. (1991). Nursing faculty practice in the Houston Linkage Model: Administrative and faculty perspectives. *Nurse Educator, 16*(5), 23–28.

Thompson, J. (1967). *Organizations in action.* New York: McGraw-Hill.

University of Kentucky (1994). *Administrative regulation.* http://www.uky.edu/Regs/AR/, retrieved from the world wide web, October 18, 2002.

University of Kentucky College of Nursing. (2002a). *Academic clinical program philosophy.* Lexington, KY: Author.

University of Kentucky College of Nursing. (2002b). *Self-study prepared for the Commission on Collegiate Nursing Education.* Lexington, KY: Author.

University of Rochester School of Nursing, http://www.urmc.rochester.edu/son/cnc/travel.html, retrieved from the worldwide Web, October 18, 2002.

Yuchtman, E., & Seashore, S. E. (1967). A system resource approach to organizational effectiveness. *American Sociological Review, 32*(6), 891–903.

Zachariah, R., & Lundeen, S. P. (1997). Research and practice in an academic communitynursing center. *Image: Journal of Nursing Scholarship, 29*(3), 255–260.

Chapter 4

Strategic Planning for Academic Nursing Practice: The Consultants' View

Bert Orlov, Lois K. Evans, Norma M. Lang, and Kathryn M. Mershon

Exemplar by Bonita Ann Pilon and Colleen Conway-Welch

An organization with a vision but no plan can be likened to a boat at sea without oars. Reaching an envisioned reality calls for a well-crafted strategic plan. Such a plan will help an organization to remain nimble and flexible while taking advantage of opportunities to meet overall objectives as they arise, respond to market forces, and refine its goals in light of a changing environment. In the challenging health care market of the 1990s—which was rife with managed care growth, consolidation, and changing provider roles—it was clear that the success of any new practice initiatives would require carefully developed strategic plans.

At the University of Pennsylvania School of Nursing (UPSON), a recently appointed dean and the faculty had worked together to develop a long-range plan for the school that built on an already strong foundation in education, research, and practice. The existing practice base comprised a partnership with the Hospital of the University of Pennsylvania, affiliations with other health agencies, and standing faculty clinician-educator clinical appointments that had been in existence for well over a decade (Fagin, 1986; see also Chapters 2 & 5). To advance the functional integration of these three arms of the tripartite mission, a clear vision was needed to drive a detailed action plan. A network of health care practices was foreseen as the practice component that would have intellectual leadership by standing faculty and clinical leadership by advanced practice nurses (APNs) and be run by UPSON. In turn, that network aimed to establish APN practice as a force in the health care market.

Academic nursing institutions like UPSON, however, had not historically employed rigorous strategic planning processes; rather, they had relied on consensus-based decision making that focused on caregiving or academic benefits, not business effectiveness. To help craft a strategic plan for the initiative, the dean sought consultation. Collaborating with UPSON's faculty and staff, the consultants introduced and applied business principles to practice development, while ensuring that the plan advanced UPSON's tripartite mission by providing new research and teaching opportunities. The consultants also worked to mediate between UPSON and the market, which viewed the initiative skeptically. This skepticism was driven by nursing's scant history as strong and visible autonomous providers within the health care system and was compounded by legal limits in Pennsylvania regarding APN scope of practice. Taken together, these internal and external challenges made this planning effort a groundbreaking initiative in health care system design.

The success of a strategic planning effort can be evaluated in two dimensions: Did the strategies work in achieving the goals, and did the planning process increase the capacity of an organization to adapt to a changing future? Based on the experience at UPSON, this chapter describes the strategic planning process in terms of internal school development and the resulting plan, evaluates both dimensions of the planning effort, and addresses some of the opportunities and barriers associated with the APN practice initiative. The importance of leadership and internal readiness to take advantage of market opportunities consistent with a school's tripartite mission are further reflected in an exemplar from Vanderbilt University School of Nursing.

UPSON PROJECT BACKGROUND AND CONTEXT

In 1991, UPSON recruited a new dean, Norma Lang, who led an internal planning process in which faculty and staff identified priorities, including further development of a practice initiative. Completed in 1992–1993, this overall plan set aggressive growth goals in student programs, research grants, practice revenues, and giving/endowment expansion. The UPSON committed to maintaining its high level of research productivity (ranked second nationally in NIH grants) and its excellence in teaching—in both the baccalaureate and the graduate programs at master's (practice and administration) and doctoral levels. For practice, the outlined vision was to create, from existing partnerships and current and potential practices of individual faculty members, an innovative array of APN practices, analogous to the medical school faculty practices (Clinical Practices of the University of Pennsylvania). Past barriers to mounting such an initiative, such as insufficient numbers of APNs and lack of research on advanced practice, had been overcome. Yet major impediments remained: insufficient financial resources and inadequate infrastructure, as well as lack of interest by faculty who viewed market-driven practice to be antithetical to nursing schools' missions and university and health-system administrators' lukewarm receptivity to the idea.

To advance this practice initiative, the dean recognized the need to develop a strategic plan that defined the APN practice goals and how to achieve them. Initial thinking focused on three areas of UPSON's strength: aging, women's health (midwifery and high-risk pregnancy), and primary care. Dialogue with colleagues in the school of medicine around potential areas for collaborative work had begun (Joint Task Force, 1993; UPSON, 1995). Because the few such previous school-sponsored practice initiatives (e.g., physician-nurse practitioner collaborative practice) had achieved only minimal success, however, the dean additionally sought advice internally and externally on new approaches. Internally, she established an ad hoc faculty committee on practice. Externally, the dean consulted with the university administration, UPSON's Board of Overseers, and APM Management Consultants, a leading health care consulting firm.

The conversation with APM Management Consultants—specifically with Connie Curran, a national leader in nursing and health care delivery and then a director at APM—led to a consulting project to develop the strategic plan. Dean Lang and Dr. Curran agreed on the value of metaresearch on APN practice and the fit of APNs in the design of innovative health care systems—a major activity of the consulting firm at that time. Conducted in 1994–1995, the consulting project developed a strategic business plan for the APN practice initiative at UPSON. The firm committed two senior consultants to conduct the project day to day: Kathryn Mershon, also a national leader in nursing and a former vice president of nursing for Columbia–HCA, and Bert Orlov, an MBA and experienced strategy consultant for health care systems and academic institutions. Both Mershon and Orlov took on the project enthusiastically and with a commitment to advance the vision espoused by the dean. Significantly, in recognition of the importance of planning within an overall context, the APM effort addressed all aspects of the school's mission. Only the practice component, however, is described here.

From a planning perspective, UPSON—as an academic institution—differed markedly from other business organizations. The autonomy of each professor/practitioner, as well as the entities of department/division/center/unit, made consensus-building uniquely essential to implementing any strategic plan. Traditionally, academic nurses have measured their success in terms of teaching, research, and *some* patient care, but without particular attention to the economics involved. Balancing the tripartite mission while meeting market and economic demands, therefore, required a process not described in the history of academic nursing. Furthermore, this initiative sought not simply to balance the elements of the tripartite mission, but rather to create a new dimension for the practice element. This initiative aimed to vivify the practice mission and create a new means of using practice to strengthen research and teaching by providing UPSON with control over a set of practices. Such control was critical to enable the use of these practices to create innovative teaching, research, and care-delivery approaches that transcended traditional nursing practice, education, and research.

To build such a practice network, UPSON had to reinvent its approach to practice development in that academic nursing differed markedly from academic medicine, with its history of business ventures. Medical schools long had lucrative faculty practice plans, joint ventures in diagnostics, and collaborations with pharmaceutical companies. Development and economic restructuring of physician faculty practice plans have had a relatively long history (see Chapter 2 and Evans, Jenkins, & Buhler-Wilkerson, 2003). During the 1980s, academic medical centers (the medical school faculties and affiliated university hospitals) had begun using consultants for strategic planning and operations reengineering. Conversely, nurses had traditionally held the status of employees rather than entrepreneurs. Consequently, nursing deans and faculty had no need to take responsibility for practice-related business planning, with its focus on revenue and profit-generation. As a result, academic nursing had less planning experience, business infrastructure, and financial resources.

In the mid-1990s, only a few small APN practices operated autonomously in the market that could offer a professional experience base on which the UPSON practice initiative could draw. Traditionally, APNs had provided highly specialized inpatient care and had led the continuing professional development of hospital nursing staff. In the outpatient setting, independently operated APN services had been limited mostly to midwifery/birthing and some primary care, particularly for the Medicaid population. As an institution and as individuals, UPSON and its faculty maintained a commitment to providing care to the underserved, making expansion of care delivery to Medicaid patients a core goal. This strategy also made market sense, because Pennsylvania was testing mandatory Medicaid managed care in Philadelphia. Hence, UPSON enjoyed a confluence of market demand, mission commitment, and patient comfort with APN services as this practice initiative began. Similarly, managed care was searching for innovative, cost-effective ways to deliver care and offered a new openness to the potential role of APNs—or, at least, the willingness to consider it.

At the outset of this planning process, the consultants assessed the market as it stood, particularly the reimbursement opportunities discovered for several existing and potential practices by UPSON faculty. At the time, most faculty directly involved in practice functioned within institutional settings, such as hospitals or visiting nurse services, where they filled APN clinical and administrative roles. Practicing faculty and APN academic support staff also participated in the teaching of students in the context of their own institution-based practice roles (see Chapter 5). Finally, several were engaged in faculty-developed APN practices, including consulting services in continence, stroke, and gerontology; a comprehensive geriatric day-hospital (The Collaborative Assessment and Rehabilitation for Elders [CARE] Program), a Medicaid adolescent health clinic, and a nurse midwifery service. Other potential practices under negotiation at the time included nurse-managed primary care practices and a multigenerational family primary-care practice. Functioning as individual faculty-led projects, these practices were not integrated with one another in any organized manner. Administrative and financial management support was limited to what the school's business office could offer based on that staff's experience with education and research. These early practices did, however, provide market experience and a starting point for developing a network with a coherent vision. In the envisioned integrated network, each of these APN practices would be linked to the school; produce standardized clinical data; share marketing, contracting, and infrastructure; and provide controlled sites for teaching and research.

Planning for UPSON's large-scale and highly visible practice initiative for APNs was novel, and the strategic planning process had three major goals. First, the process had to review and document the literature about APN practices to develop the ability to "sell" their value to the market of commercial payers (managed-care plans and traditional insurers) and their enrollees (consumers of said services, whose desire for APN care was crucial to payers' interest in APNs). Second, the practice initiative needed to marshal limited financial resources and infrastructure by tightly focusing on what populations to serve based on type of service and underlying demographics. Third, as a national leader in nursing, UPSON played an advocacy role for advancement of the profession. Therefore, success meant not only building market share and earning acceptable returns, but also setting the precedent that APNs could play an independent role within the evolving health care delivery system.

The changing health care environment, especially the then-rapid growth of managed care, presented an opportunity for UPSON to advance this professional agenda. At times, however, this professionwide agenda conflicted with the tactical imperatives for UPSON's initiative, that is, of easier entry into primary care for the Medicaid population versus reaching out to commercially insured patients. If APN care was good for everybody but the opportunity to enter the marketplace was only or mainly through Medicaid, then UPSON would have to address the implications of appearing to remain in "nursing's place" (that is, women caring for the socioeconomically disadvantaged), and, thus, "confirming" the market assumption that people who had a choice of providers would *not* consider APNs for their care.

DEVELOPING THE STRATEGIC PLAN

The strategic planning process involved both internal and external efforts, running in parallel. Within the school, among faculty, staff, and board members, the consulting project had to build the mindset that would support entrepreneurship, a market focus, and fiscally oriented management. The public nature of the planning process itself advanced this shift in mindset among the faculty. The process gave the dean and other key supporters of the practice initiative the opportunity to bring others along in supporting the vision. Equally, the process leveraged the ideas of other UPSON constituents in refining that vision. While some tenure-track, clinician-educator track, and clinical faculty and academic support staff had had experience with primary care practice, only one had run a private practice. The bulk of hands-on experience in operating practices lay in midwifery and psychiatry. Furthermore, those independent practices had operated in an *atomistic* fashion; that is, outside the school's boundaries and without institutional sanction or support (such as infrastructure or marketing).

Practitioner faculty in independent practice also faced the disdain of their more traditionally focused colleagues, who primarily valued sponsored-research and teaching and devalued practice aimed at making an economic impact on the market. As with any effort to create a new direction, those not directly involved often felt threatened because conceptions of core values appeared to be challenged and, by not being on the "inside," their stature was perceived to be potentially diminished. The planning process aimed to diminish these anxieties, which, given the nature of academic environments, could have otherwise impeded implementation of the practice initiative. Indeed, learning to think and speak in business terms—marketing/customers/pricing—presented a challenge to the faculty. For many, the language of the business of health care and of strategic planning was itself foreign at best, and indecipherable at worst. Others spoke disparagingly of this new language which, to them, appeared to repudiate the core care-giving mission of the school and of the profession. The importance of acknowledging and dealing with these two divergent paradigms cannot be overstated.

In the external (market) environment, UPSON faced the challenge of any "first mover;" that is, confronting the market with a new product that is both unfamiliar and whose value is not immediately understood. This market ignorance reflected a literal lack of knowledge about APNs as well as predispositions against more independent practice by nurses. Specifically, UPSON had to overcome presumptions about the role of physicians versus nurses, and the related *realpolitik* of the medical establishment's focus on the prerogatives of physicians. Payers reflected these views, functioning as they did within the traditional norms of physician-driven practice, in which many of their leadership positions were held by physicians. Moreover, payers had legitimate (albeit not necessarily accurate) concerns about consumer (patient) response to APNs. The combination of payer needs for greater cost efficiency and the fact of UPSON's prestige enabled the consultants to secure meetings with payer and hospital system executives previously unfamiliar with the capabilities of APNs. These discussions created a platform to introduce the value of APNs. In turn, the dialogue facilitated articulation of the "value proposition" regarding APN practice for presentation to the broader market, while helping faculty and other UPSON constituents understand how to speak to that market.

Integrating these internal (school) and external (market) efforts, the strategy development process involved three major work steps:

Step 1.   Setting the fact base about APN practice.
Step 2.   Integrating market needs with the School's vision.
Step 3.   Insuring financial and operational viability for the practice initiative.

Underlying each of these steps was work to build a foundation of support for the initiative within the school and the university at large.

Step 1: Setting the Fact Base

Mutual education was required between nursing faculty and the consultants to establish the fact base. The faculty provided insight into APN practice and how to substantiate that competency through the research and clinical literature. The consultants laid out a description of the market structure and realities of contracting, network design, and reimbursement structures. In addition, the consultants communicated the perceptions of APNs held by health care market leaders. This information created a foundation for upcoming decisions about how to focus UPSON's resources on the appropriate market sectors, based on likely patient interest and ability to secure reimbursement for independent APN services.

To begin, the consultants needed to appreciate the potential service offerings for the practice initiative. The consultants interviewed a broad range of UPSON's stakeholders, including faculty, students, staff, and members of the board of overseers (advisory to the dean) as well as leaders of the University of Pennsylvania Medical Center (medical school and hospital) and the university. Among the faculty, the consultants talked with senior and junior faculty, who represented a variety of academic (research and teaching) interests, as well as different areas of practice expertise. This range of interviews also allowed the consultants to assess the interest in and support for (or opposition to) the practice initiative.

Through these interviews, faculty shared insights about the potential roles for APNs and the research and clinical literature documenting their performance, as well as the areas of interest and expertise among the faculty. The consultants assembled and then reviewed this body of relevant literature to create the foundation for external marketing materials. The consultants documented the ability of APNs to deliver care independently, showing, for example, that 70% of primary care lies within APN scope of practice (OTA, 1986). The consultants placed particular emphasis on the contributions of UPSON's own faculty. For example, Brooten and colleagues (1986) had demonstrated the value of APNs in early discharge of very low birth-weight babies. Mezey, Lynaugh, and Cartier (1988) had demonstrated that APNs improved the health status of residents in nursing homes. And Evans and colleagues (1997) had demonstrated the effectiveness of APNs in achieving restraint reduction in nursing homes. The consulting team then relied on Mershon's administrative, business, and nursing expertise to translate these data into a framework for evaluating UPSON's potential role in the Philadelphia market.

Market context. To provide the UPSON faculty with a strong understanding of the environment within which they were designing their strategy, the consultants laid out the structures of the local and national markets and gathered information on the perception of APNs by local market leaders. These views were critical in that payers and consumers would either purchase APN services or not. While already very knowledgeable about the Philadelphia market itself, the consultants did conduct additional interviews to garner candid insights into perceptions of and potential roles for APNs. Presentations to the faculty introduced key market trends regarding how care was delivered and paid for in the rapidly growing managed care environment. Major topics included restricted networks, integrated provider systems, and the financial demands of various fee-for-service and capitation payment schemes. For Philadelphia, where managed care penetration had risen from some 15% in 1988 to nearly 30% in 1994, the market review detailed three key elements: population, care delivery networks, and payers.

- *Population:* The local and regional population was assessed in terms of geography, demographics, and payer mix (among Medicare, commercial, and Medicaid). In the geographic area surrounding UPSON, the population was largely student and Medicaid (over 33%). The consultants also sought to understand which patient populations did (not) have experience with APNs and their actual or potential reactions. Experienced with and satisfied by APN service, the Medicaid population was confirmed as a logical target for development.

- *Care Delivery Networks:* The structure and scope of integrated systems and their relative strengths were reviewed in terms of geography, clinical service, and payer class and payer-specific relationships (e.g., Independence Blue Cross and Graduate Health System). With utilization at 1,200 days/1,000 people, hospital use in Philadelphia was quite high, given its level of managed care penetration; consolidation among financially weak hospitals into larger systems seemed inevitable. The consultants also sought to understand how APNs had and could relate to those networks. Given the likely impending consolidations, a number of players expressed interest in providing innovative care and securing a link to the prestigious Penn brand.
- *Payers:* The structure and function of private and government insurance highlighted Philadelphia's highly consolidated managed care market, where only three plans (HMO of Pennsylvania, Keystone Health Plan East HMO, and HMO of New Jersey) held over 80% of enrollees. The Medicaid market was also consolidated, with Keystone Mercy Health Plan holding 60% share, and two others (Health Pass and Atlantic) holding another 34%. The consultants also sought to understand and share with UPSON those payers that had (not) and would (not) contract with and reimburse for APN practice. Success plainly required securing a deal with one of the major players.

An intersecting area of evaluation concerned Pennsylvania's plans for mandating Medicaid managed care, starting in Philadelphia. In 1993 to 1994, some 275,000 Medicaid recipients were already enrolled in HMOs, with another nearly 350,000 required to enroll over the next year. That background influenced the actions of managed care plans, existing networks, and the academic centers that historically had provided a substantial portion of the care for that population. Clearly, the growth of Medicaid managed care presented a market opportunity for UPSON's practices.

Perception of APNs. With the market context established, the consultants focused on perceptions of APNs by area payers and networks with which UPSON would need to contract or partner. Four major issues emerged: ignorance about APNs, skepticism of their value, physician opposition to their inclusion in networks, and contracting difficulties.

- *Ignorance:* Market players were not knowledgeable about APNs' capabilities in providing patient care independently or the rigorous studies demonstrating their quality. Many players still viewed nurses as physician helpers rather than as professionals competent to provide care both autonomously and also in collaboration with other providers.

- *Skepticism:* Market players doubted the willingness of patients to accept APNs as primary providers of care, except for some Medicaid enrollees and women interested in midwifery. While voicing this concern nominally on behalf of patients, the players offered no data to support (or reject) this hypothesis. Nevertheless, the perception created a barrier to integrating APNs into the networks.
- *Physician opposition:* Inclusion of APNs in networks prompted concern in the conservative East-Coast physician community for two reasons. First was the perception that nurses—even those with advanced degrees—lacked the skills to manage patient care. Second was the perceived threat to physicians' unique role in patient care and the risk of competition for patients from APNs. Even though paradoxical, these two concerns were not mutually exclusive. Nevertheless, physicians were crucial for market entry because they held the payer/network operations director positions that determined whether or not managed care organizations would contract with and reimburse APNs. In addition, it was recognized that payers and networks absolutely needed physicians, but that their relationships with physicians in general were already contentious. Therefore, physician opposition to integrating APNs into the networks appeared to payer/network leaders as presenting an additional source of conflict, which many sought to avoid. Finally, because Pennsylvania law requires physician "collaboration" when APNs practice, many physicians expressed concern regarding liability for care provided without their direct supervision.
- *Contracting:* Given the legal status of independent APNs, contracting with APNs was more difficult than with physicians. As noted earlier, Pennsylvania HMO regulations recognized only physicians as primary-care providers, thereby creating the need for physician oversight. In addition, those payers seeking partners in risk-sharing required provider networks to possess sufficient financial reserves to insure delivery of care—a problem for UPSON.

In aggregate, these four areas of challenge revealed market resistance to accepting APN practices. Even among network and payer executives who supported the role of APNs, these challenges made the inclusion of APN practices more difficult—and, from their perspective, not necessarily worth the effort.

Step 2: Integrating Market Needs with the School's Vision

In this difficult step, the priority areas for development, in planned phases, were identified. Through selecting new services to offer (by character and specialty), populations to target, and geographic areas for development, the planning process aimed to balance the interests and capabilities of the faculty with the needs of the market and its willingness to provide reimbursement for APN services. Documenting the internal capabilities of the school (as a working business system) and of the faculty lay at the heart of this step and required cultivating agreement between faculty and consultants on the basis for such measurement. The consultants had shared market information with the faculty during Step 1; because choices were now required, however, these selections were perceived as giving preference to some faculty/areas of practice over others (which was accurate—not for political reasons as feared, but because of market demands and internal skills).

Creating the strategic plan required integrating the market information with an internal capabilities assessment. Integration here means identifying overlap between realistic *market* opportunities and realistic *UPSON* capabilities. With that overlap defined, and the limits of UPSON's financial resources understood (as a limiting factor on the number of initiatives to pursue at once), the process turned to the key effort of Step 2: the selection of which services to target for development by the faculty—guided, but not forced, by the consultants. Step 2 entailed three analytical efforts, supported by a consensus-building process. First, the consultants reviewed the preliminary understanding of UPSON's capabilities against market requirements. Second, the consultants identified areas of overlap. Third, they guided the faculty in selecting target practice areas for the initial market offering. The consensus-building process addressed the faculty's limited knowledge of market requirements and business approaches to decision-making, as well as the anxieties evoked by selection of some services over others.

Analysis of capabilities and market demand. To define UPSON's internal capabilities, the consultants reviewed and evaluated the self-perceived capabilities of the faculty and UPSON (as an institution) against market requirements. The fact base completed in Step 1—and supported by the faculty—served as foundation for this evaluation of capabilities against the market standard. Clinically, the question centered on what the literature could substantiate to the market and how best to position specific practice initiatives. Each area of UPSON's clinical strength, much of it based on Penn faculty-led research—for example, primary care, midwifery, neonatology, and homecare for pregnant women, new mothers/babies, and cancer patients—represented the work of specific faculty, with their intellectual, clinical, and professional passions at play. From a business perspective, two issues arose. First, for what services would the payers/networks provide reimbursement? The answer depended, by market player, on their clinical needs and their beliefs as to where APNs could either enhance their market position or generate cost-savings. Second, the market players needed confidence that UPSON could support service delivery (requiring administrative and clinical management and infrastructure for billing), information-tracking and reporting, and quality assurance.

The consultants took the lead in conducting the internal capabilities review around these clinical, market need/interest, and business infrastructure elements. The market interviews provided the consultants with the needed insight into the views of payers/networks, thereby defining the standards against which UPSON's proposed practices would be measured. Combining this assessment of internal capabilities with what APN services the payers/networks would pay for, the consultants defined the overlap; that is, UPSON's true opportunity set. Equally significant, the consultants analyzed UPSON's financial resources. Given the limits of those resources, financing constituted a barrier to successfully mounting and sustaining a practice network and engaging in risk contracting, including capitation (see Step 3). Hence, the plan had to focus on areas of overlap as the core of the practice initiative and to make choices that limited the initial scale and scope of the planned network of practices.

Specific areas of focus for the initiative. First came the need to choose a name for the new practice initiative; the Steering Committee (see description below) settled on Penn Nursing Network (PNN). PNN's clinical priority areas were chosen based on a set of five decision criteria:

- Responsiveness to market needs in terms of available partners and opportunity to sell distinctive services to multiple payers or networks.
- Value of the service to the community and where continuity in patient services could be assured.
- Need for teaching sites for UPSON students.
- Support for research interests of the faculty.
- Financial contribution to PNN and UPSON.

Applying these decision criteria to the market assessment and internal skills review resulted in selection of service clusters for practice development. The term clusters reflected that, in the priority areas, each represented a clinical area in which multiple faculty members practiced, with overlapping yet distinctive expertise. The clusters also offered coherent programs from a marketing perspective. Three clusters were prioritized for immediate action:

- *Primary care*: Focusing on Medicaid and on targeted populations in Philadelphia under an already-obtained HRSA Division of Nursing

Multi-Generational Grant; specific practices included the Health Annex.

- *Women's Services:* Targeting nurse midwifery and the perinatal-newborn program; specific initiatives included collaboration with one or more hospital systems and managed care entities.
- *Elder Care:* Leveraging Medicare funding and combining acute and chronic care; specific initiatives included The CARE Program, gerontological consultation and continence services, and a Program of All-inclusive Care for Elders (PACE), or Living Independently For Elders (LIFE); see Exemplar, Chapter 5).

In the future, the plan envisaged creating two additional clusters. Consultative services would expand to serve as an umbrella cluster for a wide range of expertise, and a back-office service would provide coordinated contracting and billing for other faculty and affiliated practices, which were neither operating independently nor part of the three initial clusters. The plan also aimed to build a network of non-faculty APNs in practices that would link to PNN for infrastructure and/or collective marketing/contracting; in effect, an APN independent practice association (IPA), used frequently by physicians for managed care contracting).

Consensus-building process. As discussed earlier, some faculty expressed fear that the decision making about which services to develop involved more politics than business logic—that the selections were preordained and/or driven by the dean's or select faculty member's personal preferences. Knowing from the outset of the project that such political issues swirl in academic environments and could prevent effective planning and support for implementation, the consultants recommended—and the dean established—a highly participatory process for the strategy development effort. Information sharing with the faculty focused on business planning and market functioning, on the consultants' findings regarding how the market judged APN capabilities and value, and on what constituted realistic market opportunities. Thus, the faculty came to appreciate that the market defined some services as more viable than others, based on payer reimbursement and patient demand, and that market requirements did not necessarily dovetail with areas of clinical or research excellence.

In actuality, this consensus-building process had already begun at the start of Step 1, when the consultants had interviewed a broad range of UPSON's constituents. In addition, at the start of Step 1, a faculty steering committee had been established—and announced to the faculty. This committee's role was to work with the consultants and make a formal recommendation regarding the plan to the faculty senate, which had the power to approve or reject the plan. The committee's members brought diverse perspectives for decision making, sufficient seniority and prestige to carry weight with other faculty (in effect, as spokeswomen for the practice initiative), and representation of the key practice skills that would be deployed in the market. This new, separate committee was needed to focus on an integrated strategy, reaching across the traditional boundaries of research, teaching, and practice. Its role would become central to project beginning in Step 2, when difficult decisions about priorities would have to be made.

Throughout Step 2, the consultants (and faculty) presented findings and proposals to the steering committee. Typical of strategic planning processes, subgroups from within the steering committee were created to act as work groups. By initially reviewing findings and strategic options, these work groups leveraged the time of the steering committee and included additional faculty in the dialogue, thus expanding the reach of the process and securing further skills and input. Focused on different clinical specialties, each work group met weekly to review the findings of the consultants and provide reaction/input to the strategic options developed by the consultants. Based on these discussions, the consultants transformed options into concrete "straw-woman" models to which faculty/practitioners could react further, prompting the iteration of the straw-women into increasingly focused and compelling proposals. It was at this stage that the steering committee became involved, through its monthly meetings, in providing broader feedback on the straw models to focus ongoing refinement and develop consensus.

To extend the consensus building, each work group's faculty leader sat on the steering committee, giving each group a champion within the planning structure and within the faculty at-large. To build support among the entire faculty, the consultants and key steering committee members interfaced with the existing faculty committees. In addition, the consultants conducted several open sessions for the entire faculty to keep them informed of, and provide opportunities for input into, the evolving strategic plan.

Step 3: Insuring Financial and Operational Viability for the Practice Initiative

To implement the plan, UPSON needed an economically driven approach to the allocation of its limited human and financial resources. Issues of concern included anticipated patient volumes, expected reimbursement levels, provider productivity and compensation, and development of settings for practice, including space and staff. UPSON also needed to create an internal organization, which was not in place at the time. The plan laid out this structure and leadership roles, as well as the professional status of and internal relationships needed to support and manage the practitioners as members of a larger nursing care network. Equally significant, the plan detailed the required infrastructure systems for functions such as billing, scheduling, credentialing, and facility management, as well as recommendations on how to secure them. In business argot, the three options here were to "build" capacity internally *de novo*, "use" (or, rather, leverage) capabilities within the entire university, or "buy" through vendor contract or joint venture with outside companies (see more detailed discussion in Chapter 7; Swan & Evans, 2001). These decisions depended on internal expertise, relative costs, and importance of direct control over given functions.

Based on targets established in Step 2, the consultants developed financial and organization plans for PNN. They proposed targets for revenue and expense (including start-up costs) for each planned practice. In parallel, they also outlined possible organizational structures for management and oversight as well as for infrastructure. The steering committee reviewed the consultants' proposals, recommended modifications, and selected a strategy. These decisions reflected the political realities of the academic environment and the financial constraints of UPSON's resources. Overall, the organizational model called for a single coordinated administrative structure for management and clinical control. Administrative operations were designed to coordinate all the PNN practices into a coherent network facing the market. PNN aimed to create a shared systems/process infrastructure, supported by sharing of profits and prorata overhead contribution by each practice. The plan also called for a routine annual process for budgeting and performance review, overseen by the faculty.

Organizationally, the model represented a hybrid between traditional academic structures and a business model. Academically, the director of academic nursing practice was to be a member of the standing faculty, reporting directly to the dean with a line to the UPSON Faculty Committee on Practice. This director would have responsibility for day-to-day management of the clinical operations of PNN, specifically the recruitment/retention of qualified APNs and their clinical performance. Coordinating with the director (where appropriate), a nonclinical chief operating officer (COO) would have responsibility for developing the practices, building the infrastructure, running marketing/contracting, and leading budgeting and financial oversight, as well as day-to-day management of sites/staff and systems/infrastructure. Administrative duties would include quality assurance/utilization review, site operations, financial performance (including revenue and expense management), care delivery processes, human resource management (for the staff, not the clinicians) and coordination with the faculty leaders of education and research initiatives in each practice. The external relations dimension of the COO's role were to focus on marketing, contracting, and customer service, as well as on legal issues and purchasing. In the initial development of the infrastructure, the COO was to coordinate development of required administrative capabilities, such as payer negotiations, contract management, liability and benefits, and computer services for operations, finance, and clinical data management. Together, the director and the COO would report to the dean and work with the proposed standing faculty committee on practice.

Comprising faculty and senior staff, the committee on practice was to have membership paralleling the diversity of the strategic planning steering committee, such that the committee on practice could function as liaison between the practice initiative and the faculty as a whole. Routine responsibilities included ongoing strategic planning and regular reviews of performance. Annual goal setting involved more comprehensive review of performance, as well as budget approval. For each practice, specific performance indicators were reviewed, including clinical quality, financial performance (against budgeted expectations), and patient service and mission support; that is, the quality of the educational opportunity (and teaching) and support of research initiatives, including effective data sharing.

EVALUATION OF STRATEGIC PLANNING PROCESS

As already noted, the effectiveness of a strategic planning process can be measured against the degree to which the plans helped meet organizational goals and the degree to which the organization developed new capabilities. Some of the ample evidence for both of these achievements is detailed here.

Effectiveness of Planning

The strategic planning process served its central objective: The PNN became a reality. Opportunities were selected from each cluster, and practices were either established or initiated, according to the plan. Overall organization and infrastructure development also went forward largely as planned, with some modifications based on PNN size and budgetary restrictions.

For the primary care cluster, PNN opened and has operated since 1995 a community-based nursing center in a building annexed to a city recreation center; the Health Annex provides integrated primary care, mental health, and women's health services (Reed, 1997; see also Chapter 11). Serving primarily a Medicaid managed care population, the Health Annex helped focus and force action on the issues regarding access to APN services: that is, need for regulatory change in regard to the definition of primary care provider in the HMO laws, licensure, and prescriptive privileges, and direct reimbursement (Jenkins & Torrisi, 1995; Lang, Sullivan-Marx, & Jenkins, 1996; Jenkins, 2002; Sullivan-Marx, 2000). Many other challenges provided grist for the mill in learning about the real world of providing access to APN services in an academic setting. These included contracting with various managed care companies, maintaining collaborating physician arrangements and staff stability, marketing to achieve and sustain adequate enrollments, and overcoming relative isolation from the university community. The evolution of the Health Annex also provided unprecedented opportunities for developing new models of community-academic partnerships in support of research, education, and practice (see Chapter 11). Through the Health Annex, PNN has also been able to play a major role in the National Nursing Centers Consortium (NNCC). Membership in NNCC has enabled PNN to seek jointly regulatory change to ensure financial viability of nursing centers (see Chapter 12) and participation in the development of a shared nursing center database that will be critical for research and policy change (see Chapters 8 & 9).

In the area of women's health, PNN found that women did indeed seek nurse midwifery services in those sections of the city where PNN established its practice base between 1995 and 1999. One of the major lessons learned was about the politics of contracting with health systems and hospitals for admitting privileges. The second was about competing for Medicaid patients with obstetrical residency programs in a marketplace where, simultaneously, the birthrate was rapidly declining and Medicaid payment rates were being dramatically reduced. Using the strategic plan as a guide, PNN was able to make projections about long term viability. The PNN and faculty leaders were able to conclude that these practices would not be viable in the foreseeable future and made the difficult but financially necessary decision to phase them out. The research-based perinatal newborn program provided a special opportunity to learn about working with commercial managed care. This service, and one based on the same model for a chronically ill population, became options for negotiations by the university's technology transfer office. Although the service was never fully operationalized, based on the resultant delay and the payer's programmatic changes, the licensed home health agency that was developed for it was transitioned to LIFE (see later), thus supporting the early development of another PNN practice.

Practices in the elder care cluster have proved perhaps the most successful for PNN, in large part because of both lower competition in the field and the evolving synergy and strength of the UPSON gerontologic faculty in all three areas of education, research, and practice (see Exemplar B, Chapter 5). The CARE Program had many positive outcomes, such as development of a computerized patient record that included a nursing classification system (see Chapter 8), operating a Medicare comprehensive outpatient rehabilitation facility (CORF), developing collaborative relationships with colleagues in medicine and other fields, and training hundreds of students in interdisciplinary team care. The decision process that was used to close this practice after six years closely adhered to the protocols developed in the strategic plan, helping PNN correctly frame the decision in terms of external environmental issues—in this case, the effects of the Balanced Budget Act of 1997 (Evans & Yurkow, 1999). Experience with all of the gerontologic practices provided a base for initiating LIFE, a PACE program certified by Medicare and Medicaid to provide integrated primary, acute, and long-term care services to an enrolled set of frail nursing-home eligible community-residing elders (Naylor & Buhler-Wilkerson, 1999). Assuming no major reductions in capitation rates, LIFE is projected to be financially successful. The experience of the CARE Program and LIFE have provided unique opportunities for PNN, the nation's first and only school-of-nursing network to have operated either a CORF or a PACE program.

Recognizing that, like any practice, the "ramp up" to full productivity/revenue-generation would take time, PNN phased in its organizational structure and infrastructure services. A business manager/chief financial officer was hired in 1994, and a tenured faculty member was appointed to the director of academic nursing practice (DANP) position in 1995. The overall operations responsibilities were shared between these two positions until 1998, when an associate director for operations (similar to the proposed COO) was appointed. As PNN closed practices, thereby generating less revenue for infrastructure, this position was abolished in 2000 and the DANP and others reabsorbed the related duties. PNN has continued to use the model for infrastructure development (make, use, buy), with shifts occurring as PNN became more sophisticated or practice needs changed (Swan & Evans, 2001; see Chapter 7). Many of the functions originally envisioned as taking place centrally, for example, are now being managed at the practice level due in large part to the very diverse nature of each of the practices requiring distinct processes for billing, collections, contracting, quality management, credentialing, and information systems (see Chapter 7).

During startup of the network of entrepreneurial practices, fiscal resource needs were managed in various ways. Most new practices enjoyed some grant funding initially (see Table 6.3 in Chapter 6) while building a client base; grants were also secured in support of some of the infrastructure development, notably the clinical information system (Marek, Jenkins, Westra, & McGinley, 1998; see also Chapter 8). Fee-for-service, capitation, and other insurances and contracts contributed increasing amounts to the bottom line. To meet startup requirements for LIFE, as well as to provide support during early development for other practices, UPSON also negotiated access to a line of credit from the University of Pennsylvania. Inviting university administrators to join school advisors, faculty, and staff in a Financial Oversight Group for Practice (FOGP) provided ongoing opportunities to educate and influence the greater university about the value of PNN services for the school, the university, the community, and the society (see Chapter 6).

The academic organizational structure was implemented essentially as laid out in the strategic planning process. In 1994, UPSON did not have a standing committee on practice. Based on the strategic plan, the faculty bylaws were amended to create such a committee, chaired by the DANP. Continuing to the present, the practice committee has developed new ways for the school at large and the practice network and infrastructure to interface and insure effective communication and mutual understanding. Facilitating a broad conceptualization of academic practice for UPSON, the practice committee has also highlighted the contributions of the clinician-educator faculty and other faculty who practice with joint appointments, as well as the school's partnerships and affiliations with health care entities. Sponsoring an annual series of academic practice rounds, for example, has been one way the practice committee has focused attention on integration of the tripartite mission (see Chapter 9). The criteria for decision-making about new practices and goal-setting for existing practices within PNN has remained in use. Finally, the framework for evaluating practices has grown into an annual report card. The faculty director and practice director for each PNN practice is required to report to the practice committee regarding goal achievement, both in terms of the tripartite mission and also the business operations, including quality.

Organizational Capacity Building

In general, a combination of the newness of the initiative to the market, the relative managerial inexperience of practice leadership, and micro- and macroeconomic and political challenges played a role in how PNN actually developed. The strategic plan proved useful, however, as PNN worked systematically to carve out niches in the three cluster areas. The focus on remaining nimble and flexible was a new concept in the academic environment; thus, knowledge and awareness of the market helped frame decisions to open, close, merge, or transition practices as appropriate (see also Chapter 5, Table 5.2). As described earlier, UPSON was able to make opportunistic (and difficult) decisions in a timely fashion. For example, new services were opened when a payment source became available (Hamburg, LIFE). Conversely, practices were closed when market and/or reimbursement streams were no longer viable (The CARE Program, Perinatal Newborn Program, Continence, the two nurse midwifery services). Also practices were merged for economies of scale (Health Corner with Health Annex, the two midwifery services), and transitioned to another practice (home care license to LIFE) to save time and expense of redevelopment.

UPSON's ability to take these types of decisive actions underscores the importance of consensus building through an input-driven and representative structure. Nevertheless, in reality, there will probably never be total agreement about a school-owned practice initiative. This result is hardly surprising. Institutional change is a long-term process. Slower than envisioned growth reflects health care macroeconomics (competition from physicians and consumer demand for provider choice) and the challenges that nursing has faced since the late 1990s, in Pennsylvania and nationally. These factors have contributed to the limits of its embrace by UPSON stakeholders.

The strategic planning process itself provided UPSON with several demonstrable benefits, with the clearest measure of success being the actual implementation of the plan for launching PNN. As for process, the consultants helped to set the dual foundation of pragmatism about the market and of a reasonable level of internal support. This foundation—which is now far stronger than at the project's outset in 1994—has enabled PNN to operate and continue moving forward, despite setbacks. The strategic planning framework has endured, helping PNN (through its director and the practice committee) to focus on selected priorities and to evaluate strategy and performance (by practice and overall) on a regular basis.

The framework has also continued to provide clear measures of success and for decision making. Finally, the plan itself, for its strengths and weaknesses, provided a basis for taking action: PNN was created, and there is no substitute for "learning by doing." While generally true, the importance of learning by doing cannot be overstated here, given that this effort represented the first-ever attempt to create a network of independently operating APN practices that made an impact on the market at large.

LESSONS LEARNED

From the perspective of innovation, the very act of creating the PNN—a network of nursing practices analogous to a medical school faculty practice plan or integrated outpatient network—constitutes a breakthrough in health care system design. As the first effort to create such a network of APN practices, PNN has created a framework on which future APN and other nursing initiatives can build. The following discussion addresses lessons learned from PNN's experience.

Cash is Queen. Ongoing cash flow (through profits or a line of credit) is needed to ensure the ability of a start-up initiative to weather reversals and continue to market and develop the network. This marketing/network effort focuses on gaining patient volumes and operating effectively, thereby making a case for support—or, at least, the need to be acknowledged by—major systems or payers. This point underscores the importance of starting with clear backing from the university, a major health care system, or payer as a prerequisite to launching such an initiative. (As an aside, PNN may well have enjoyed greater success by deferring launch until its leadership had secured such support for the PNN entity. However, waiting may well have prevented the ultimate launch of an integrated network, thereby precluding any experiential learning.)

What worked. The PNN strategic plan created success by beginning with vision, leadership, and communication, then moving through concrete elements of the strategic planning framework. First, PNN came into being because the dean and faculty shared a vision for a network of practices that would influence health care in the market, for the good of patients, and for nursing (Lang, 1996). Moreover, Dean Norma Lang made a personal and public commitment to push the agenda, even against market resistance, physician objections, and internal skepticism. Furthermore, the dean had the courage to seek outside expertise to supplement internal skills and experience. Leadership also came from the director of academic nursing practice and other faculty who believed in the initiative and worked for its development. Their diligence proved critical, from planning through implementation—at times tedious and even painful, as when a practice had to be shuttered. Together, the consultants supported the dean and the faculty champions to develop an internal process for consensus building and communication. This operational framework built a core of support and then advanced the cause of the initiative, as seen in the ongoing strength of the organizational structure designed for PNN.

A key element of consultants' contribution lay in leading the strategic planning process, grounded in market and financial realities. This expertise, based on experience, was limited among the UPSON faculty, but it was critical for making a credible attempt at building a business, particularly one as novel and complex as PNN. Reaching out to payers and networks, as potential partners and sources of guidance for developing the initiative, was also critical, and the consultants played a key role as credible and independent liaisons. Had the Philadelphia market not consolidated as it did between 1995 and the present, some of those contacts may have delivered real results. For example, the hospital system most excited about collaboration with UPSON—and which happened to serve a substantial Medicaid population—ended up being absorbed by another system, less keen on collaboration.

Based on these observations of the strategic planning process at UPSON and the history of PNN, several lessons can be offered for other nursing networks under development. Four key points warrant focus:

1. Start with a vision and committed leadership—both at the top and for the day-to-day management of the practice network—to leverage with the research and educational components of the mission.
2. Reach out to the market, and involve numerous players (internal and external) to get the best advice and most innovative ideas on how to organize, focus, and market the practice network.
3. Be ruthless in dealing with business realities—even though that approach may be countercultural in some academic environments.
4. Ensure that there are adequate financial resources (working capital) for launching practices and funding the requisite infrastructure and marketing initiatives.

In summary, a combination of market interest, perceived quality, and available resources defines the extent to which a network of APN (or any other practices)—as distinct from stand-alone initiatives—can become significant market players. As one of the first such initiatives, PNN achieved a modest level of success. PNN offers a model for the next group of nurses who enter the health care market with dual goals of caring for patients and transforming the role of nursing. An organization that has a clear vision and organizational and operational readiness can take advantage of market opportunities (see also Exemplar). Such activity in the marketplace advances the professional agenda for nursing and can thereby strengthen the health care system by providing new options for and approaches to care delivery.

Exemplar.
Vanderbilt University School of Nursing and the TennCare Program.

TennCare is Tennessee's state-managed Medicaid program, established in January 1995. It has over 1.4 million enrollees statewide. At the time TennCare was initiated, Vanderbilt University School of Nursing (VUSN) was operating a small primary care clinic in an underserved Housing and Urban Development (HUD) project using nurse faculty providers. In addition to family nurse practitioner primary care services, the Vine Hill Community Clinic provided mental health services delivered by faculty psychiatric-mental health specialists. Originally funded by a grant from the W.K. Kellogg Foundation (1991), the clinic was operating on a financial base that included Medicaid fee-for-service (FFS), sliding-scale collections, and Medicare. Viewed essentially as a clinical laboratory for students and a faculty practice site, the clinic's primary aims did not include generating a positive cash flow; indeed, deficits were covered by VUSN's operating budget.

As the state and the medical center struggled to switch from FFS Medicaid to managed Medicaid in early 1995, it became apparent that there were few viable primary care venues within the Vanderbilt University Medical Center (VUMC). The School of Medicine and its residency programs were very much specialty based. There was no family practice residency program. The medical center found itself looking for way to handle a managed Medicaid population with few physician resources. VUSN was ideally positioned within the Medical Center to absorb the growing Medicaid population and to do so in a clinically sound, cost-effective way. Since the mid-1990s, the Vine Hill Community Clinic and its nurse faculty providers had been a significant source of care for the Medicaid enrollees for whom VUMC was now at financial risk.

In 2001, VUSN providers subcontracted 8000 enrollees from VUMC for primary care. The clinic receives a primary care subcapitation payment on a per-member per-month basis. Other revenue is generated by Medicare payments, sliding-scale self-pay, and some commercial insurance; TennCare capitation payments, however, constitute 95% of the clinic's revenue base. FY 2002 saw more than 15,000 patient visits. In 1988, the clinic had added prenatal services with deliveries at Vanderbilt Hospital, using faculty who are certified nurse midwives (CNM). Approximately 55% of births are TennCare referrals from the primary-care population cared for at the Vine Hill Community Clinic. In FY 2002, the midwifery service attended just over 200 births. Patient satisfaction with nurse managed care remains high.

Since its early days, Vine Hill Community Clinic and the other practice sites have come to be viewed by the entire VUSN faculty as more than just clinical placement sites for the academic program. Increasingly, faculty view the practice network as a valuable resource for research and model testing in advanced practice. Concomitantly, the practice program has been charged with achieving financial sustainability without relying on school of nursing operating funds. In the past two years, the practice program at Vine Hill has improved its financial results from a deficit to a surplus. The midwifery program has achieved breakeven status and is experiencing unprecedented growth, doubling its volume every 12 months. Approximately 350–400 births are projected for FY 2003.

The strategic alliance with TennCare and with the medical center has greatly facilitated the growth and sustainability of VUSN's faculty practice program. Clinical outcomes and utilization measures demonstrate improvement over conventional medical care for this population. As the state struggles with possible changes in TennCare, VUSN keeps in close contact with the MCOs to determine how best strategically to align the goals of its program with future funding opportunities.

—Bonita Ann Pilon and Colleen Conway-Welch

REFERENCES

Brooten, D., Kumar, S., Brown, L. P., Butts, P., Finkler, S. A., Bakewell-Sachs, S. et al. (1986). A randomized clinical trial of early hospital discharge and home follow-up of very low birthweight infants. New England Journal of Medicine, 315, 934–939.

Evans, L. K., Strumpf, N. E., Allen-Taylor, S. L., Capezuti, E., Maislin, G., & Jacobsen, B. (1997). A clinical trial to reduce restraints in nursing homes. *Journal of the American Geriatrics Society, 45*(6), 675–681.

Evans, L. K., Jenkins, M., & Buhler-Wilkerson, K. (2003). Academic nursing practice: Implications for policy. In M. D. Mezey, D. O. McGivern, & E. Sullivan-Marx (Eds.), *Nurse practitioners: Evolution of advanced practice* (4th ed., pp. 443–470). New York: Springer.

Evans, L. K., & Yurkon, J. (1999). Balanced budget act of 1997 impact on a nurse-managed academic nursing practice for frail elders. *Nursing Economic$, 17*(5), 279–282.

Fagin, C. (1986). Institutionalizing faculty practice. *Nursing Outlook, 34*(3), 140–144.

Jenkins, M., & Torrisi, D. (1995). Nurse practitioners, community nursing centers, and contracting for managed care. *Journal of the American Academy of Nurse Practitioners, 7*, 1–6.

Jenkins, M. (2002). Abbottsford community health center and Pennsylvania politics. In D. J. Mason & J. K. Leavitt (Eds.), *Policy and Politics in Nursing and Health Care* (4th Ed.), pp. 87–91. Philadelphia: Saunders.

Joint Task Force on Primary Care Pilot Programs (1993, July 30). *Proposal from the Joint Task Force of the School of Medicine and the School of Nursing on Primary Care Pilot Programs*. Philadelphia: Author.

Lang, N. (1996). Academic nursing practice: A case study of the University of Pennsylvania School of Nursing. In *Penn Nursing: The Publication of the University of Pennsylvania school of Nursing, 1*(1), 17–19, 36.

Lang, N. M., Sullivan-Marx, E. M., & Jenkins, M. (1996). Advanced practice nurses and success of organized delivery systems. *American Journal of Managed Care, 11*(2), 129–135.

Marek, K. M., Jenkins, M., Westra, B. L., & McGinley, A. (1998). Implementation of a clinical information system in nurse-managed care. *Canadian Journal of Nursing Research, 30*(1), 37–44.

Mezey, M., Lynaugh, J., & Cartier, M. (1988). A report card on faculty practice: The Robert Wood Johnson Teaching Nursing Home program, 1982–87. *Nursing Outlook, 36*, 285–288.

Naylor, M. D., & Buhler-Wilkerson, K. (1999). Creating community-based care for the new millennium. *Nursing Outlook, 47*(3), 120–127.

Office of Technology Assessment (1986). *Nurse practitioners, physician assistants, and certified nurse-midwives: A policy analysis* (Health Technology Case Study 38, OTA HCS-37). Washington, DC: U.S. Government Printing Office.

Reed, D. (1997). The development of a community-based nurse managed practice network by the University of Pennsylvania School of Nursing. In *The Third National Primary Care Conference Case Studies*, pp. 229–140. Washington, DC: HRSA.

Swan, B. A., & Evans, L. K. (2001). Infrastructure to support academic nursing practice. *Nursing Economic$, 19*(2), 68–71.

Sullivan-Marx, E., Happ, M. B., Bradley, K. J., & Maislin, G. (2000). Nurse practitioner services: Content and relative work value. *Nursing Outlook, 48*, 269–275.

University of Pennsylvania School of Nursing (Feb. 27, 1995). *School of Nursing Network and Penn Health System*. Presentation to Penn Health System Implementation Group. Philadelphia: Author.

Chapter 5

Making Academic Nursing Practice Work in Universities: Structure, Function, and Synergy

Lois K. Evans, Maureen P. McCausland, and Norma M. Lang

Exemplars by Patricia Chiverton and Neville E. Strumpf

A school's appreciation for its own history, mission, and internal and external environments is critical for achieving academic practice success (Evans, Swan, & Lang, 2003; see Chapter 3). As the University of Pennsylvania School of Nursing (UPSON) began to expand its academic practice agenda in the early 1990s, several contextual strengths and limitations could be identified. For example, an existing and strong entrepreneurial value within the university encouraged the development of new businesses. The school had a critical mass of faculty scholars and clinicians for mounting such an initiative. Yet UPSON's status as the only school of nursing within an ivy-league university to have all three levels of nursing education posed a challenge for university administrators in finding relevant benchmarks. Further, the university's strong emphasis on research meant that efforts to build a practice agenda would need to be couched within that framework.

The school's colocation on a single campus as one of 12 autonomous schools, which included four health professional schools and an academic medical center, provided a precedent for a rich environment as well as role models for health care activities as part of the academic mission. Strong disincentives for cross-school activities existed, however; chiefly, concern over sharing indirect cost recovery, tuition revenues, and leadership. Moreover, the school's autonomy from the university's academic medical center was a double-edged sword in that it could also limit access to considerable practice-relevant resources. The school's ability to harness strengths and manage limitations would be pivotal to its success.

This chapter is focused on the model of academic nursing practice at UPSON with particular attention to its development over the past decade. Model, mission, and component structures and functions are described. Emphasis is placed on the ways in which mission synergies—a desired outcome—were achieved through leveraging planned expansion of the academic practice mission. Exemplar A illustrates a synergistic and complementary relationship between the University of Rochester School of Nursing and its university health system, and Exemplar B exemplifies the synergies that can occur when all three arms of the tripartite mission are well structured and developed in a particular area, gerontological nursing at UPSON.

STRUCTURING ACADEMIC NURSING PRACTICE

In most schools of nursing, standing faculty teach and carry out scholarly activities. An expectation for practice requires careful consideration of how faculty roles are defined, how the faculty functions, and how faculty members are promoted and rewarded. Also needing serious consideration is how the school organizes itself to carry out its major functions. Even in institutions that value clinical faculty roles and where other professional schools have had a long history of implementing practice agendas, the announcement by a school of nursing that it intends also to fully operationalize and integrate its tripartite mission will produce reverberations within and without.

For one thing, schools of nursing are capitally deprived as compared with their medical, dental, and law school peers. For another, academic nursing is just now achieving its stride in generating funded research, long a hallmark of great universities; a resurgent emphasis on practice, it is feared, will take away energies and resources from the research agenda. Academic nursing's typical operational separation from nursing service (see chapter 2) has meant less experiential knowledge of managing health services. Too, nurses did not have access to reimbursement for their clinical services until recently; in hospitals today, payment for nursing care is neither separate nor distinct from the daily hospital rate, even while evidence mounts of its critical importance to patient care outcomes. The impact on changing such paradigms of prevailing perceptions about "women's place" and "nursing's place" is legend. Finally, academic nursing has tended to follow the university mental model and, thus, to have a different orientation from that required to manage and deliver health services on a 365-days-a-year (365) and 24-hours-a-day, 7-days-a-week (24/7) basis. Each of these facts may give pause to both schools of nursing and to their parent institutions contemplating new futures that involve academic nursing practice.

ACADEMIC NURSING PRACTICE AT UPSON

Practice integrated with research and education is integral to the mission of UPSON (see Chapter 1). Academic practice at UPSON has three major components (see Fig. 5.1). These are the practices of individual faculty, particularly those of the clinician educator faculty; practices accessed through partnerships and alliances with health care organizations including the University of Pennsylvania Health System (UPHS), Children's Hospital of Philadelphia (CHOP), Visiting Nurse Association of Greater Philadelphia (VNA) and others; and practices of the school-owned Penn Nursing Network (PNN). Within each of these components, interdisciplinary collaboration is emphasized.

The school's academic practices could be described as a mixed portfolio, representing a range on the ownership, performance, and clientele continua (see Fig. 3.2 in Chapter 3). The most recent component to be developed is the school-owned practice organization—the Penn Nursing Network (PNN). Previously, UPSON had enjoyed more than a decade of jointly appointed standing faculty in administrative, research, and advanced practice leadership positions in its own hospital (Hospital of the University of

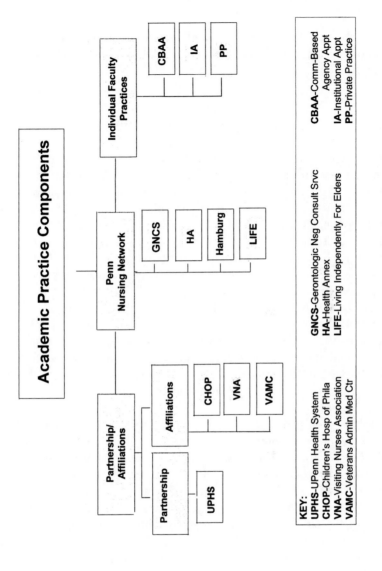

Academic Practice Components

Partnership/ Affiliations

Partnership
- UPHS

Affiliations
- CHOP
- VNA
- VAMC

Penn Nursing Network
- GNCS
- HA
- Hamburg
- LIFE

Individual Faculty Practices
- CBAA
- IA
- PP

KEY:
UPHS-UPenn Health System
CHOP-Children's Hosp of Phila
VNA-Visiting Nurses Association
VAMC-Veterans Admin Med Ctr

GNCS-Gerontologic Nsg Consult Srvc
HA-Health Annex
LIFE-Living Independently For Elders

CBAA-Comm-Based Agency Appt
IA-Institutional Appt
PP-Private Practice

FIGURE 5.1 Model of Academic Nursing Practice at the University of Pennsylvania School of Nursing.

Pennsylvania [HUP]), CHOP, and elsewhere. Each component of the school's academic practices is briefly described to explicate relevant structure, function, governance, and management.

Practices of the Faculty

Many standing faculty at UPSON are engaged in practice-related activities, which range from providing direct clinical or administrative services to providing education and/or conducting research in academic practice settings. Clinician educators (CE) are members of the standing faculty who spend a designated portion of their time in clinical practice. For the majority of CEs at UPSON, a contract with a clinical agency is used to specify the time, role, and salary/benefits arrangements. Tenure-track faculty may practice as well, and some have negotiated a practice component to their Penn role, particularly when it relates closely to their program of research; a few others have maintained "moonlight" practice appointments (see Chapter 3). Generally, however, practices of the faculty refers to those practices that faculty members (primarily CEs) have tailored so as to play an integral and synergistic role in their scholarship and teaching. All CEs are engaged in bringing the best evidence-based practice to the bedside (see descriptions in Chapter 10), and from this base their own scholarship evolves.

In the 1980s, the newly approved CE role (Clinician-educator track, 1984; see also Chapter 2) gave impetus to renewed innovative trials of collaborative physician-nurse faculty practice initiatives; like their earlier predecessors, these had a mixed history of success, especially in collaborative primary care and nurse midwifery practices with faculty from the school of medicine. Smaller "projects" with evaluation components such as those funded through Mary Rockefeller grants more often were sustained (e.g., Wanich, Chapman, Mezey, Lavizzo-Mourey, & Medford, 1990). Two additional programs conducted during the same period gave visibility and prestige to UPSON's academic nursing practice initiatives. These were the national Robert Wood Johnson Teaching Nursing Home Program (TNHP) that was managed by the school and the Robert Wood Johnson Clinical Scholars Program (CSP) for which the school served as a training site. The TNHP project demonstrated on a national basis the importance of linking schools of nursing with nursing homes, especially through jointly appointed advanced practice faculty and staff, for achieving overall improved care and resident outcomes (Mezey, Lynaugh, & Cartier, 1988; Shaughnessy, Kramer, Hittle, & Steiner, 1995). The CSP launched doctorally prepared nurse clinicians on interdisciplinary clinically focused research careers and helped to underpin further the school's commitment to clinical scholarship and research.

The CE role has been vital to all the health professions schools at the University of Pennsylvania (nursing, medicine, dentistry, veterinary medicine, and social work) in that it places major emphasis on scholarship of *practice* and teaching, as compared with the emphasis, for tenure-track faculty, on *research* and teaching. In each of the two roles, scholarship remains an important component, but may be operationalized differently (see, for example, Chapter 10). The definition of scholarship for the two tracks has been differentiated by the faculty in its appointment, retention, and advancement criteria; further, practice is one component considered in the merit review process.

At UPSON, a balance of tenure-track and clinician-educator appointments is assured through a limit (since the early 1990s) of appointments to the CE track to 40% of the total number of standing faculty. Of 16 faculty holding CE positions, nine are at UPHS, four are at CHOP, and one each is in three other settings. Two of these CEs hold major administrative leadership positions in their respective agencies, while others are in expert clinical leadership positions. Because of their breadth and depth of experience, the CEs have provided much leadership and support for PNN as well, including quality management consultation, clinical information system development, advanced nursing practice, and faculty academic leadership. In addition to Nursing Research and Administration, professorial titles of CEs include cardiovascular nursing, community health nursing, gerontological nursing, geropsychiatric nursing, health care of women, medical nursing, nursing of children, nurse midwifery, nutrition sciences, oncology nursing, primary care nursing, psychiatric mental health nursing, psychosocial nursing, trauma and critical care nursing, and women's health nursing. Practice roles or positions are negotiated jointly by the faculty member and division chair, together with the dean and with agency leadership. For the practice component of the role, the CE is accountable to the contracting agency; for teaching and scholarship components, to the division chair in the UPSON.

A large number of part- and full-time advanced practice nurses, some doctorally prepared, function as academic support staff and are integral to the school's classroom and clinical teaching mission. Many of the full-time APNs also enjoy jointly appointed practice positions in a range of settings, including the PNN and partner/alliance agencies, thus further adding richness to the tripartite mission at UPSON.

Partnerships and Alliances

Like leading schools across the country seeking to establish more formal links with nursing service in their university-owned hospitals and medical centers, UPSON developed in the early 1980s a partnership model with its medical center (Hospital of the University of Pennsylvania–HUP). This arrangement acknowledged the different but complementary missions and agendas of nursing at each institution and provided for appropriate linkages that would enhance the shared agendas in research, education, and excellence in clinical care (Fagin, 1986; Chapter 2). Notwithstanding its pros and cons, the model has survived the test of time and continues to facilitate important relationships between the two institutions.

Commensurate with approval of the CE role in 1983, faculty appointments were made jointly between the school and HUP and with other clinical agencies that would formally link the relevant entities. A faculty position (clinician educator) in UPSON—associate dean for practice—was created for the chief nursing officer at HUP. At its inception, this associate dean and professor of nursing administration role was focused primarily on maintaining excellence in nursing service at HUP, facilitating educational experiences for nursing students and access to settings and populations for faculty and doctoral student research. It also enhanced synergies between the two organizations by jointly appointing faculty and clinicians to committees, credentialing faculty for practice in the HUP, teaching nursing administration and leadership, and advising on curriculum and standards. In the early period, most of the clinical directors at HUP also held CE faculty appointments.

While no formal documents were generated that linked the Children's Hospital of Philadelphia with UPSON, clinician-educator faculty have consistently been appointed to leadership and advanced clinical practice roles there as well, beginning also in 1983. More recently, similar appointments for faculty have occurred within the VNA (VNA; Buhler-Wilkerson, Naylor, Holt, & Rinke, 1998). Efforts to forge standing faculty appointments at the Veterans Administration Medical Center of Philadelphia have been unsuccessful to date because of the challenges of federal appointment rules.

Since the middle 1990s, HUP has been part of a large integrated health system, UPHS, whose other components currently include three additional hospitals, faculty and community-based physician practices, home care, hospice, and nursing home. When this expansion was initiated, UPSON faculty strongly recommended a position at the system level for a chief nurse executive (CNE) who would also serve as associate dean for practice at the school. The implementation of this position gave nursing a place at the table for corporate decision-making that affected the quality of, and environments for, professional nursing practice throughout the system. As HUP took its place as one of several entities in the system, CEs held fewer administrative leadership but maintained clinical leadership positions at HUP; to date, no positions in other components of the UPHS have been filled by CEs. Adjunct and clinical faculty titles for incumbents in several system hospital nursing leadership positions have been used, however, to link the institutions with the school. At CHOP, administrative leadership (associate director for practice and research) and clinical leadership appointments (e.g., endocrine clinical nurse specialist, pediatric nurse practitioner, lactation specialist) have continued relatively unchanged.

University of Pennsylvania Health System

Since UPHS is a formal partner with UPSON, detail about its nursing service structure is provided. At UPHS, the CNE leads the design and testing of the professional practice model (McCausland, 1997). This model was first evolved at HUP and has now been institutionalized in nursing service systemwide. The chief nursing officer at each system hospital and the CNE are together accountable and responsible for the standards of nursing practice, nursing education, and nursing research wherever a nurse practices. The senior leadership team is rounded out by doctorally prepared and expert leaders who chair nursing's systemwide governance committees (e.g., nursing practice and ambulatory care, advancement and recognition, research, product evaluation and standardization). The governance system is inclusive and participatory, with committee representatives from each hospital also serving on the system-wide committees. A strong and decentralized management structure contributes to maintaining environments that support professional practice.

Research utilization, evidence-based practice, and interdisciplinary collaboration are highly valued components of nursing at the UPHS. The three types of variables that are used to measure the success of the practice model are structural (e.g., educational preparation of nurses, turnover and vacancy rates), process (e.g., physician-nurse collaboration, patient satisfaction scores, Press-Ganey nursing scores), and outcome (e.g., alterations in skin integrity, falls with injury, urinary tract rates, pain management, interdisciplinary outcomes).

Having a professional practice model in place makes nursing service settings in UPHS extremely important to the education of undergraduate and graduate students; such a rich environment is also supportive to collaborative research. Jointly conducted searches for clinician educator faculty to serve in key leadership and clinical positions in UPHS have been an important strategy for achieving these goals. Tenure-track faculty and the dean have also, over the years, supported the professional practice model through serving on a variety of UPHS and hospital committees (e.g., trustees, research) and providing in-service education. Likewise, UPHS clinical leadership and staff often serve as adjunct faculty or academic support staff in the school, teaching and/or serving on task forces and committees.

Practices of the Penn Nursing Network

Background. While CE practices and strong clinical affiliations provided rich resources for academic practice at UPSON, there was growing recognition of the need for academic community-based services, especially in nurse midwifery, gerontological nursing, and primary care. The strategic planning that preceded the launching of PNN, UPSON-owned practices, is described in detail in Chapter 4. For illustrative purposes and because much of the content of this book refers to the issues surrounding school-owned practices, attention is given here to the mission, structure, and operation of this component of UPSON's academic practice portfolio.

Mission and vision. Building on the schools' strategic plan to "lead the profession through demonstrating best practice approaches and roles for nursing in a rapidly evolving healthcare market" (UPSON, 1995b, Nov. 10), PNN was formalized in 1995 with faculty leadership and a small infrastructure. The PNN mission and vision, congruent with that of the UPSON, are found in Table 5.1. Table 5.2 highlights PNN practices over a decade (see also Chapter 4 for a more detailed description). Designed to be nimble and flexible in order to take advantage of market opportunities and trends, as well as respond to educational and research needs, practices were opened, closed, or merged as warranted, following application of criteria developed as part of the strategic plan (see Chapter 4 for a discussion of rationale for these decisions).

Established criteria for opening new practices (see Chapter 4) include that they meet a community need, have likelihood continuity, meet school needs for education and research programs, and are fiscally sound. Each practice is evaluated annually by the practice committee; fiscal health is assessed on a monthly basis (see Financial Oversight Group for Practice [FOGP] below; Chapters 4 & 6 describe outcomes of PNN practices).

TABLE 5.1   Penn Nursing Network Mission and Vision

Mission Statement. Penn Nursing Network (PNN), a multipractice health care delivery network spanning the life cycle, is committed to community-based health care of the highest standard. PNN embraces health as a cornerstone for quality of life as defined by the person and supported by PNN staff. PNN promotes proactive health care, fostering active participation and personal responsibility in health care decisions.

PNN adheres to the belief that quality health care is defined as the degree to which health services for individuals and populations increase the likelihood of desired health outcomes and are consistent with current professional knowledge. Such outcomes are achieved through partnership with individuals, families, and the community and the integration of research-based practice, education of professionals and community members, and scientific inquiry. PNN is committed to quality health care that is cost effective, utilizing the most advanced and appropriate healthcare models and interventions.

Vision Statement. PNN seeks to provide individuals, families, and the community with respectful and confidential quality care while educating healthcare professionals, developing research-based practice guidelines, and maintaining economic stability. PNN strives to improve health services to the community and is committed to affirm this vision with the care of each individual (UPSON, 1999).

Faculty governance. The development of PNN was guided by the strategic plan, goals, mission, and vision as established by the faculty; business plans for each practice; and an organizational structure (see Chapter 4) that included a position for a director of academic nursing practice reporting directly to the dean and a standing committee on practice of the faculty senate. The practice committee has several related functions: to examine the practice missions of UPSON and PNN, to advise the dean and faculty senate on policies related to academic practices, to monitor the internal and external environments and their potential impact on the academic practices, to provide a forum to examine practice issues and make recommendations to the faculty as appropriate, and to review proposals for the development of new academic practices (UPSON, 1996).

Several deliberately crafted elements serve to link PNN intimately to the school's mission. Faculty ownership and governance are assured through the practice committee, chaired initially by the director for academic nursing practice (and later co-chaired by the associate dean for practice). Both clinician-educator and tenure-rack faculty sit on this committee, as do the faculty academic director and the director for each practice. While the practice committee oversees and provides guidance to the overall practice mission of the school, it also provides particular oversight for

TABLE 5.2 Overview of Penn Nursing Network Practices FY 1995–2002

Practice	Description	Period of Operation	Clients Served	Education	Scholarship	Comments
The Collaborative Assessment and Rehabilitation for Elders (CARE) Program	Nurse-managed geriatric day hospital providing intensive rehabilitation services. Certified as Medicare CORF	FY 1993–1999	Total = over 700 frail elders with complex health and rehabilitation needs	Total = 641 nursing & interdisciplinary students	6 research studies; 9 publications	Closed by UPSON following implementation of BBA '97 that reduced reimbursement by > 70%.
Community Midwifery	A women's health and full scope nurse-midwifery service with offices at Health Annex and Health Corner	FY 1995–1999	X 38 births per year; culturally diverse, mostly MA insured	X 7 students/ year		Merged with Neighborhood Midwifery (1999) for efficiency; closed by UPSON FY99 due to changes in market & reimbursement.

TABLE 5.2 *(continued)*

Practice	Description	Period of Operation	Clients Served	Education	Scholarship	Comments
Continence Program	Nurse-managed non-surgical continence interventions in ambulatory and long term care sites	FY 1988–2002	X 513 encounters/year. Older adults, culturally diverse, mostly Medicare insurance	X 12 students/ year	3 research projects; 6 publications	Placed on inactive status in 2001 when faculty expertise no longer available and market changed
Germantown Midwifery	Contract start-up midwifery service in community hospital	FY 1996–1997	n/a	2–4		Hospital preferred to open own service and did not renew contract; GM evolved into Neighborhood Midwifery

(continued)

TABLE 5.2 *(continued)*

Practice	Description	Period of Operation	Clients Served	Education	Scholarship	Comments
Gerontologic Nursing Consultation Service (GNCS)/ PNN Consulting	Education and consultation by advanced practice nurses and other professionals focused on research-based care for older adults and other areas, including academic nursing practice	FY 1988–current	Over 120 advanced practice nurse and interdisciplinary consultants providing average 95 services/year			Important research dissemination vehicle for faculty. Has remained successful by attending to market trends and opportunities in a range of areas. Closely linked to Hartford Center of Geriatric Nursing Excellence
Hamburg Center	Women's health services. Contract with the PA Department of Public Welfare	FY 1997–current	X 135 encounters/year. Women in a residential center for adults with developmental disabilities	1–2 students/year		Half day/month practice.

TABLE 5.2 (*continued*)

Practice	Description	Period of Operation	Clients Served	Education	Scholarship	Comments
Health Annex at the Francis J. Myers Recreation Center	Primary care community nursing center providing integrated health, mental health, women and men's health services. Located in a neighborhood recreation center	1995–current	In FY 2001: 2,209 primary care encounters; 19,066 outreach encounters [includes Health Corner] culturally diverse community	FY 2001: 59 students, 5,516 hours	6 research projects; 12 publications	Reimbursement from MA capitation and other insurance, FFS, contracts for family planning, immunizations and other services, grants; incorporated Health Corner in 2000
Health Corner	Primary care, gynecologic, family planning, teen and women's health services. Located within a community center	1984–current (a satellite of the Health Annex)	[see Health Annex for data]		1 publication	Began as a clinical education site for graduate students, developed an adolescent/family planning service, and later evolved into a satellite for Health Annex providing women's health and primary care

(*continued*)

TABLE 5.2 (*continued*)

Practice	Description	Period of Operation	Clients Served	Education	Scholarship	Comments
Keeping Teens Healthy	Specialized integrated health and psychosocial program to promote successful transition from middle school to high school	FY 1994–1996	Vulnerable middle school students in low income area		1 research project	Funded project ended; no reimbursement available from usual funding streams
Living Independently For Elders (LIFE)	Certified Program of All-inclusive Care for the Elderly (PACE) providing 24/7 integrated acute and long term care services	FY 1998–current	At FY 2001 108 members enrolled; frail older adults who are nursing home eligible and prefer to live in the community	FY 2001 57 students, nursing & interdisciplinary	1 research project; 1 publication	Fully certified Medicare/ Medicaid Program of All-inclusive Care for the Elderly (PACE) program

TABLE 5.2 *(continued)*

Practice	Description	Period of Operation	Clients Served	Education	Scholarship	Comments
Perinatal Newborn/Home Health Services	Specialized, research-based in-home advanced practiced nursing service to promote healthy start for low birth-weight infants; certified Medicare home health agency.	FY 1996–1997	High risk mothers and their infants			Research-based practice, certified as home health agency; developed in collaboration with commercial insurer for its members, but closed when market changed

(continued)

TABLE 5.2 (*continued*)

Practice	Description	Period of Operation	Clients Served	Education	Scholarship	Comments
Neighborhood Midwifery	Women's health and midwifery services. Collaboration with LaSalle Neighborhood Nursing Center and a private practice	FY 1997–1999	Grew to 18 births/year	2–4	1 study	Evolved from Germantown Midwifery; unique collaboration with another community nursing center; incorporated Community Midwifery in 1999 before being closed by UPSON due to changes in market and reimbursement

programmatic and quality aspects of the PNN practices. For each practice in PNN, a faculty academic director (one or more standing faculty members, either tenure track or CE, who take leadership for a particular practice) provides the overall intellectual leadership, vision, and direction for the practice model to be employed; facilitates educational and research activities; and sets the research agendas. Further, the faculty academic director secures and maintains outside funding for start-up and special programs associated with the particular practice.

The director for academic nursing practice position was first filled in 1995. This standing faculty position (the initial incumbent was a tenured faculty member) reported directly to the dean and is responsible for facilitating operational, fiscal, and quality outcomes for the tripartite mission within the entire network of practices. The position also has responsibility to direct, facilitate, and represent broadly the practice mission of the school. The position was vacated during FY 2002, and the functions were shared by the faculty academic directors and the associate dean for practice while the faculty complete a revision of UPSON's overall strategic plan, including its vision for academic nursing practice.

Management and operations. Day-to-day management for PNN practices is provided by advanced practice nurses (APNs) or administrators; these directors sit on both the practice committee and the FOGP (see below), and they meet regularly with the director of academic nursing practice as the PNN Leadership Group. The APNs, and other clinicians as appropriate to the particular practice, provide the services. These may include—but not necessarily—clinician educator faculty.

Revenues for the PNN practices are primarily patient revenues (Medicare and Medicaid, both fee-for-service and capitation; commercial insurance; managed care capitation, out-of-pocket), service contracts, and public and private grants and gifts. In addition, the university granted UPSON a line of credit to serve as startup capital. An aggressive growth projection for PNN initially envisioned total revenues of $10 million by FY 2000; in actuality, the numbers are tracking but delayed by about three years (see Chapter 4).

Operations and fiscal advisement and management are achieved through several mechanisms. The FOGP (see Chapters 1 and 6) is an advisory group to the dean on the fiscal health of PNN. It comprises members of the school's volunteer board of overseers who hold particular expertise in the business of health care, university administrators, and outside advisors, together with key administrative personnel in the PNN infrastructure (see Chapter 7) and the school. This group has helped PNN and UPSON to develop a level of sophistication in its fiscal management for practice that provides assurances to leadership at all levels. Each practice is guided in its ongoing development and operations by an executive committee and finance subcommittee that meet on a regular basis; the chair of the finance subcommittee represents the practice on the FOGP. The practice directors and school business administrators meet as a PNN Business Group.

Evolution of PNN infrastructure has been commensurate with the changing size and sophistication of the network of practices (see Chapter 7). Currently, functions specific to the needs of a particular practice are being managed at the practice level, reserving responsibility for overall financial, development, and information systems management (see Chapters 8 & 9) at the central infrastructure and/or UPSON level; payroll, human resources, legal, risk management services are obtained through the university. Using an allocated cost formula, an indirect charge is levied against each practice to support infrastructure and cover costs to the UPSON central services and university that accrue from PNN. At the University of Pennsylvania, each school and unit is expected to operate on a balanced budget; thus, PNN and each individual practice must also balance its budget each year.

SYNERGISTIC OUTCOMES ACHIEVED IN UPSON'S TRIPARTITE MISSION

Synergy Through the CE Role

Clinician educator faculty have been key to achieving synergy in advancing academic nursing practice at UPSON. Bringing the real world of practice to the classroom, the state of the science knowledge for best practices to the clinical area, and questions that still need answered to the research arena remain important to UPSON and its partner/alliance agencies. The relationships developed between CEs and other practitioners, both nursing and multidisciplinary, help foster the development of a community of scholars in these agencies (Riley, Beal, Levi, & McCausland, 2002). UPSON's early adoption of the CE role at the standing faculty level was critical, especially in a research-intensive institution, for maintaining respect for the "scholarship of practice" within the university community. Because all are prepared at the doctoral level and are appointed to the rank of assistant professor or above, they also enjoy greater opportunity to compete for extramural funding for projects, including research, which adds credibility to their important role within the school and university. Examples of synergy achieved through appointment of clinician educators are described in Chapter 10.

Synergy in Research-Practice Teams

Fagin (1986) once predicted that academic "practice designs that do not reflect the research agenda are doomed from the start" (p. 144). The PNN strategy of planning a research agenda as part of the model for each practice was built on this truth. It has been the case for the CEs as well, who have developed research practices or carved out research from their practice (e.g., O'Sullivan & Jacobsen, 1992; see Chapter 10). The synergy achieved by working collaboratively with other nurse and interdisciplinary researchers (especially through the partnership/alliance agencies) has yielded greater outcomes than any one scholar could likely have accomplished alone. Examples of such research teams are found in the work on transitional care in a variety of populations, with initial work having been conducted by CE and tenure-track faculty at HUP and UPHS (e.g., Brooten et al., 2002). This work also demonstrates the importance of recognizing where value is being placed, both within and outside the institution, and of positioning ongoing effort so that it can be supported to meet a range of goals.

Synergy in Leadership

Initially, the associate dean for practice and the director for academic nursing practice each reported separately and directly to the dean concerning their specific accountabilities, the former primarily in regard to the school's linkages with UPHS and the latter primarily for development and operation of PNN and leadership for the overall academic practice mission for the school. Over time, as greater stabilization occurred in the newly formed UPHS and in PNN, convergence between the roles and goals of the two could be observed. The incumbents worked together to develop the strategic plan for practice for UPSON and to co-chair the committee on practice. The associate dean for practice took responsibility for working with the CEs in their scholarly practice development, while the director for academic nursing practice assumed overall responsibility for PNN practice development and outcomes and codirected the office for research in academic practice (see Chapter 9) with the director of the center for nursing research. Together they implemented strategies that would meet mutual goals for advancing academic practice, such as cosponsorship of academic nursing practice rounds. Other strategies were related to sharing areas of expertise across systems, for example, specialized knowledge about credentialing, quality assurance, best practices; identifying common areas for scholarly practice development, knowledge building, and translational research in support of evidence-based care; and exploring common nursing sensitive quality indicators for tracking across multiple settings.

Synergy in Partnerships and Alliances

The partnership with nursing at UPHS serves a vital role in support of UPSON's tripartite mission through excellence in nursing practice, commitment to the education and socialization of future practitioners, and support for and participation in the research mission of the university. The alliances with other partners serve similar functions. Such alliances also offer a rich environment for integrating the tripartite missions of the school. Continuing development of these affiliations, alliances, and partnerships should focus on meeting mutual goals related to research-based practice and clinical education. These might include the development of a set of common data elements to facilitate research across practices.

Synergies with Research Centers

As described in Chapter 9, synergy between the school's research centers and academic nursing practice settings has been slow to develop. Probably because of the close match between practice and center, a notable exception is the Center for Gerontologic Nursing Science/Hartford Center of Geriatric Nursing Excellence (see Exemplar B). Linking centers from the inception of planning for a new practice initiative may be an effective way to co-join strengths of each, helping to establish the research agenda and database that will be required to sustain it. Follow-up think tanks, research seminars, availability of pilot grants, and shared academic nursing practice rounds may, when available consistently over time, yield greater synergies for practice-based research. Further, evidence exists of the value in developing practice-based research networks (Deshefy-Longi, Swartz, & Grey, 2002); this concept could be used well in an academic practice model spanning as broad a range as that of UPSON, linking nursing practices in similar settings across multiple settings. Such an opportunity already exists for PNN's Community Nursing Center through its affiliation with the National Nursing Centers Consortium (see Chapter 12).

Synergy in Learning

Practices of the faculty, those in the partner/alliance institutions, and those in PNN provide unique living laboratories for integrated health care practice, research, and education. Students and faculty alike have enjoyed unprecedented experience in the business of nursing and health care, especially through PNN, and a joint UPSON–Wharton School graduate program in nursing administration recognizes the value of executive leadership preparation for nursing practice. Nursing faculty have gained a legitimate place at the table with physician faculty and other health care players. Service learning opportunities abound, through PNN especially, as faculty and students provide community service in and develop enduring relationships with the school's West Philadelphia community. Efforts to achieve a fully integrated model have given wide national and international circulation of the Penn Nursing brand.

CONCLUSION

Nursing has had a long presence on the University of Pennsylvania campus. This history itself, however, continues to shape some of its current challenges and context (see Chapter 2). After a decade of intense investment in community-based academic practice development, built on a strong base of clinician-educator faculty practice and partnership/alliances with health care institutions, UPSON is now engaged in another strategic planning period in which it will reexamine this mission along with its others. Like any organization, the more the school can ascertain where it is now, the better able it will be to move forward in these times of uncertainty and ambiguity. Pausing to reflect on the following lessons learned about structure, function, and synergy is critical to decision making about the next steps:

- *Relationships are key.* Important relationships have included those with the dean; between the associate dean for practice and director for academic nursing practices; between faculty and other clinicians, interdisciplinary colleagues, students, and overseers; between the school and the community; and between the school and university and health system administrators.

- *Research integration is hard work.* It is also dependent on such factors as the degree of control over the practice environment, having a critical mass, stability in practice systems, and practical considerations (see Chapter 9).
- *Unanimous support for academic nursing practice is unlikely.* If one waits to begin until total consensus is reached, the first step will never be taken and the goals never achieved. A critical mass is all that is required.
- *Academic practice must be fiscally responsible and sustainable to be successful.* Plans for supporting loss leaders deemed essential to the mission must be developed.
- *Dynamic tension between vision and operations is a given.* Administrative leaders and faculty must develop a degree of comfort with ambiguity.
- *Staying open to seeing patterns and making predictions in times of uncertainty and ambiguity is extremely difficult.* This is especially true when the times are turbulent (as when major change is occurring, either within or without; that is, rapid conversion from fee-for-service to managed care models, rapid growth in disparate models without sufficiently stable infrastructure, or closure of practices or programs owing to reimbursement or market changes (see Chapter 4). During the 10-year period described here, HUP/UPHS experienced such turbulence as it formed a new entity and endured a rapidly changing health care market, as did PNN as it opened and closed or merged several practices in a three-year period. In such environments, it is easy for day-to-day survival to take precedence over the larger goals.
- *Flexibility is a challenge when a school assumes long-term responsibility for standing faculty.* Education, research, and practice resources must be leveraged carefully to support key faculty and staff through rapidly changing times.

Yet, as Bennis and Biederman (1997) remarked, "The ability to plan for what has not yet happened, for a future that has only been imagined, is one the hallmarks of leadership of a great group" (p. 40). For UPSON, if past academic leadership is prologue, then the school can only anticipate a unique future for its integrated tripartite mission.

Exemplar A.
University of Rochester School of Nursing, Community Nursing Center.

The Unification Model that integrates nursing education, practice, and research is the hallmark of the University of Rochester School of Nursing (URSON). This model was established in the early 1970s under the leadership of Dean Loretta Ford and was first implemented with joint appointments for faculty who also practiced in the hospital setting. In the late 1980s, a community nursing center was created that expanded the concept of joint appointments to a community setting. This move led to increased visibility for URSON and supported the concept of nursing faculty as independent practitioners.

As the University of Rochester's Health Care System continued to expand, the role of URSON within an academic medical center became less clear. While the school contributed to the education and research missions of the medical center, the practice link was missing. Joint appointments continued, but the school did not participate in setting the strategic direction for the health care system. A new dean was inaugurated in 2000 and negotiated the additional position of vice president for nursing for the health care system. The deans of nursing and medicine report to the vice president and provost for health affairs and participate on the senior management team for the health care system. The collaboration that occurs during management team meetings identifies opportunities for the community nursing center to participate in health care system initiatives. URSON now contributes to the entire tripartite mission of the academic health center.

With unlimited opportunities for expansion, the Community Nursing Center faculty identified a focus of health promotion as the umbrella for business initiatives. An entrepreneurial business was created that not only added value to the health care system but also generated revenue for URSON. This entrepreneurial nursing model is distinct from the prevailing medical model. Both models are interdependent. Neither owns the other. Neither is defined by the other.

One of the first business line initiatives was the purchase of a travel health franchise called Passport Health. The medical center already had two travel clinics run by physicians that met one day a week. With the *support of the health system leadership team, URSON opened the Passport Health Clinic; the other medical center clinics closed, and the two physicians became the medical directors of the URSON clinic.*

Another example of the value a school can add to a health care system occurred when the weight management center was moved from the department of medicine to the school of nursing. Weight management fits under the umbrella of health promotion and consists primarily of nutrition and nursing interventions. Because of the complexity of the hospital system, the clinic was mired in bureaucracy, and the staff was unable to quickly make the change required to establish a profitable weight management program. One of the benefits of starting an entrepreneurial business line in the school of nursing is the ability to be flexible and to respond quickly to changes in the market place. This clinic staff now participates in many of the health care system initiatives, and the program is a profitable business.

One of the most exciting initiatives for the community nursing center was the creation of a health promotion program. Health promotion interventions are, for the most part, nursing interventions. The faculty in the community nursing center conceptualized a new model of care called Health Checkpoint that integrates technology and nursing interventions. The technology provides a "real time" connection with the consumer in the community. The program has a patent pending and is being licensed to a corporation for national distribution. URSON will receive royalties from this program that will fund new education or research initiatives. This model of care not only promotes the health of the Rochester community, but also offers a worksite wellness program to its own health care system, another value added by the school of nursing.

Through the creation of diverse lines of business, URSON is able to generate revenue that supports new education and research initiatives. If one business line has difficulty performing, as did the Passport Health Program after September 11, 2001, the other lines of business offset the losses. Schools of nursing across the country are experiencing fiscal challenges as they strive to demonstrate, to university finance officers, a return on investment. Tuition reimbursement and research dollars do not support the infrastructure of many schools of nursing. As a result, many nurse educators find themselves in a position of financial jeopardy. The creation of a faculty practice not only generates revenue for a school, but also adds value to the health care system as a whole.

—Patricia Chiverton

Exemplar B.
Achieving Synergy in the Tripartite Mission:
The Case of Gerontologic Nursing.

Deeply influenced by the early leadership of Claire Fagin, Mathy Mezey, Doris Schwartz, and Joyce Colling, gerontologic nursing represents the integration of the tripartite mission to a greater degree than in any other specialization at the University of Pennsylvania School of Nursing (UPSON). Under the umbrellas of the Center for Gerontologic Nursing Science (CGNS), and, later, the John A. Hartford Center of Geriatric Nursing Excellence (HCGNE), UPSON has now achieved synergy far beyond previous dreams through its interrelated programs of research in individualized and transitional care for frail elders and special aging-related clinical problems; academic nursing practice in acute, long-term, and community-based settings demonstrating innovative models of care for frail older adults; and strong baccalaureate, masters, doctoral and postdoctoral educational programs in gerontologic and geropsychiatric nursing. Such visible integration evolved over time through insightful and sustained faculty leadership; development of a critical mass of scholars, clinicians, and educators; and collaborative work with physicians and other interdisciplinary colleagues.

By 1980, a masters-level gerontologic nurse clinician program (GNP) was in place at UPSON, followed mid-decade by a required gerontologic theory and clinical course for undergraduates and integrated geropsychiatric theory and practice in the graduate psychiatric-mental health nursing program. Postdoctoral training support was available by the late 1980s. Further, in collaboration with the school of medicine, nursing faculty codirected the Geriatric Education Center, which aimed at preparing interdisciplinary teams for geriatric practice. These educational and training programs enjoyed support from HRSA, NIMH, and NIA.

Simultaneously with the development of its educational programs, UPSON moved rapidly, through strategic clinical faculty and preceptor appointments and leadership by a senior level clinician educator (CE), to create novel (at the time) roles for APNs in practice programs, including comprehensive geriatric assessment; collaborative team practice in outpatient, nursing home, and home-based primary care; and nurse-managed services such as continence care and poststroke consultation. Most of these were in interdisciplinary practice settings that involved physician faculty in geriatrics from Penn's School of Medicine. The Ralston-Penn

Center for Geriatric Education and Care, and, later an institute on aging, aided in the development of interdisciplinary practice, education, and clinical research. That gerontologic nursing and geriatric medicine developed in parallel at Penn undoubtedly played an important role in the ability of UPSON to assume and maintain coleadership in practice, education, and research development.

Beginning in 1993, UPSON took the lead in opening and operating selected specialized practices for the frail elderly, including The Collaborative Assessment and Rehabilitation for Elders (CARE) Program and a Program of All-inclusive Care for the Elderly (PACE, or Living Independently For Elders–LIFE), both components of the Penn Nursing Network (PNN). A research agenda for these practices ensured that clinical data would be available for outcomes evaluation and multiple studies. Similarly, clinician educator faculty with appointments at the Hospital of the University of Pennsylvania (HUP) carved out practices in geropsychiatric liaison nursing and otorhinolaryngology linked to faculty scholarship and clinical placements for undergraduate and graduate students.

Concurrently, programs of gerontologic nursing research for frail elders were also being developed, the two earliest of which were individualized, restraint-free care and transitional care, followed by programs in sleep, end-of-life care, acute confusion, depression, trauma, caregiver skill, health outcomes, and decision sciences/telehealth. A critical mass of researchers in these and related areas grew such that today, 18 standing faculty and 12 adjunct faculty are associated with the CNGS/ HCGNE. In 2002, 13 doctoral students and 5 post doctoral students at UPSON have made a commitment to careers in gerontological nursing science. In addition, 3 endowed professorships and 2 term chairs were held by gerontologic faculty, further leveraging mission integration. Aiding in the dissemination of the faculty's research findings, the Gerontologic Nursing Consultation Service (GNCS) has, since 1988, provided expert advanced practice education and consultation. Part of the PNN, the GNCS has been instrumental in helping to shape standards of practice for elders in nursing homes and hospitals.

Faculty leadership has been essential in garnering and sustaining the critical mass of scholars, clinicians, and educators in gerontological nursing that UPSON enjoys today. In recognition of its strengths, the John A. Hartford Foundation designated UPSON as one of five Centers of Geriatric Nursing Excellence in the United States. Based on a 20-year history, the center is dedicated to building the science of geriatric care, developing and testing innovations, disseminating best practices, and educating the next generation of clinicians, scholars, and leaders (http://www.nursing.upenn.edu/centers/hcgne).

—*Neville E. Strumpf*

REFERENCES

Bennis, W., & Biederman, P. (1997). *Organizing genius: The secrets of creative collaboration*. Reading, MA: Addison-Wesley.

Brooten, D., Naylor, M. D., York, R., Brown, L. P., Munro, B. H., et al. (2002). Lessons learned from testing the Quality Cost Model of Advanced Practice Nursing (APN) Transitional Care. *Journal of Nursing Scholarship, 35*(4), 369–375.

Buhler-Wilkerson, K., Naylor, M., Holt, S., & Rinke, L. (1998). An alliance for academic home care. *Nursing Outlook, 46*(2), 77–90.

Clinician educator track in the School of Nursing (April 13, 1984). *University of Pennsylvania Almanac, 4*(5).

Deshefy-Longi, T., Swartz, M. K., & Grey, M. (2002). Establishing a practice-based research network of advanced practice registered nurses in Southern New England. *Nursing Outlook, 50*(3), 127–132.

Evans, L. K., Swan, B. A., & Lang, N. E. (2003). Evaluation of the Penn Macy Initiative to Advance Academic Nursing Practice. *Journal of Professional Nursing, 19*(1), 8–16.

Fagin, C. M. (1986). Institutionalizing faculty practice. *Nursing Outlook, 34*(3), 140–144.

McCausland, M. P. (1997). Professional Practice Model. In *Nursing Service Policy Manual*. Philadelphia: University of Pennsylvania Health System.

Mezey, M., Lynaugh, J., & Cartier, M. (1988). A report card on faculty practice: The Robert Wood Johnson Teaching Nursing Home Program, 1882–1987. *Nursing Outlook, 36*, 285–288.

O'Sullivan, A., & Jacobsen, B. (1992). A randomized trial of a health care program for first time adolescent mothers and their infants. *Nursing Research, 4*(4), 210–225.

Riley, J. M., Beal, J., Levi, P., & McCausland, M. P. (2002). *Journal of Nursing Scholarship, 34*(4), 383–389.

Shaughnesssy, P. W., Kramer, A. M., Hittle, D. F., & Steiner, J. F. (1995). Quality of care in teaching nursing homes: Findings and implications. *Health Care Financing Review, 16*(4), 55–83.

University of Pennsylvania School of Nursing (February 27, 1995). *School of Nursing Network and Penn Health System*. Presentation to Penn Health System Implementation Group. Philadelphia: Author.

University of Pennsylvania School of Nursing (November 10, 1995b, rev.). Strategic Plan. Philadelphia: Author.

University of Pennsylvania School of Nursing (May 6, 1996). Bylaws. In *Faculty Manual*. Philadelphia: Author.

University of Pennsylvania School of Nursing (November 15, 1999). Penn Nursing
    Network Mission and Vision, revised. *Minutes of the Practice Committee*. Philadel-
    phia: Author.
Wanich, C., Chapman, E., Mezey, M., Lavizzo-Mourey, R., & Medford, A. (1990).
    Continence services for the ambulatory elderly: A comparison of geriatric nurse
    clinician (GNC) and GNC-MD team managed care (abstract). *Gerontologist,
    30*(Special Issue), 44A.

Part **II**

Resources and Strategies for Implementing Academic Practice

Chapter 6

Strategies for Securing Business Expertise, Financial Support, and Visibility

Norma M. Lang, The Honorable Marjorie O. Rendell, Jeffrey S. Levitt, Catherine R. Judge, and Susan Greenbaum

Exemplar by Susan Greenbaum

sking for help is an important strategy for success and growth. A well-conceived model and business plan for establishing school-owned academic nursing practices must include strategies for identifying and cultivating advisors, securing funds, and achieving visibility through public and media relations. University or school board members, financial and other senior university administrators, consultants, community supporters, friends, donors, and the media can each play an important role in achieving viability of academic nursing practices. Each expert participant brings some part of vital financial, business, policy-making, fundraising, and public relations expertise that can help leverage and advance the goals of the school and its practices in key ways. Once participants understand and embrace the academic nursing practice mission and its strategic importance to improved health care, these business, health care, academic, government, and community leaders can be among a school's greatest advisors, advocates, and ambassadors (Lang & Evans, 1999). Such involvement and participation may sound easy on the face of it. For schools of nursing unaccustomed to identifying and evaluating the realities of owning and operating Academic Nursing Practices—and the business imperatives that drive those practices—assembling and building key alliances, such as those described in this chapter, can mean the difference between setting sail in a canoe and in a catamaran.

This chapter considers how the creation and cultivation of a board of expert advisors and "friends," together with the use of fund-raising and public relations or marketing techniques, can strengthen the viability, visibility, and success of an academic nursing practice enterprise. Examples from the experiences of the University of Pennsylvania School of Nursing's (UPSON) Penn Nursing Network (PNN) are presented to demonstrate key points.

BUILDING COALITIONS OF ADVISORS AND CHAMPIONS

Finding the right advisors requires thoughtful matching of program needs with the talents and resources of the experts sought. There are volunteers waiting to be asked to help. The best leaders are those who come to understand and share a school's passion and vision. They should have complementary skills and resources, be able to fill gaps in faculty and staff expertise, and have the time to devote to intensive advisory sessions. A school's existing governance and its parent university's senior administrative structures can be among the first and most obvious groups to draw on. Those regents, trustees, board members, senior vice presidents, and chief academic officers allow schools to capitalize on sophisticated administrative and volunteer leadership systems already in place within the academy. UPSON is fortunate to have such voluntary expertise in a board of overseers.

Board of Overseers, UPSON

While the trustees have overall governance and fiduciary responsibility for the academy, each of the 12 schools within the University of Pennsylvania has its own presidential and university trustee-appointed board of over-seers. In addition to the chair—usually a trustee or other loyal alumnus—the university's president and trustees appoint 25–30 overseers to advise and advocate for the school. Each individual school is responsible for deciding priorities for, and how it will make use of, its board. Within UPSON, overseers advise on all goals of the school, including education, research, practice, fundraising, communications, diversity, international-ization, and physical and financial resources. Overall practice goals and achievements are on the agenda at all overseer meetings each year. In addition, overseers are selected to serve on governance or advisory commit-tees for individual practices as well as on a general oversight group for practice. While overseers are concerned with all programs of the school, in this chapter, only the academic practices are addressed.

Financial Oversight Group for Practice

Drawing on its board of overseers and other expertise, UPSON created a special Financial Oversight Group for Practice (FOGP) for the purpose of advising the dean on all business aspects of PNN, the school-owned aca-demic practices. The FOGP was established at the same time that the university advanced the school a line of credit, which UPSON had requested to support the start-up of selected PNN practices (see Chapter 4). Because UPSON did not have a long history of operating academic practices, experi-enced business leaders were sought for FOGP membership who had the health care, business, financing, marketing, and policy expertise to help UPSON's academic practice leaders successfully monitor and navigate the financial and health care markets. Several overseer members who had been serving on the individual governance bodies for three of the PNN practices, and, in some cases, chairing a finance subcommittee for a specific practice, were natural choices to be asked to serve on the FOGP when it first was formed. In addition to those overseers chosen for their particular expertise, members outside the school of nursing came from the University of Penn-sylvania's current and former senior leadership, including the vice president for finance, the controller, and the provost or chief academic officer. Within the school, members included the dean, vice dean for administration and finance, director of academic nursing practices, associate dean for practice, and several others.

Members of the school's board of overseers were asked to join the FOGP as a strategic matching of overseers' talents to the needs of the school. The

FOGP provides an effective, positive way to tap into overseers' interests in and enthusiasm for particular aspects of the school's mission—practice, of course, being key among them. These and other community and business leaders provide an endorsement for PNN practices (and school as a whole) that adds important weight to the expertise of faculty and staff. Carefully choosing members of the FOGP also is critical to a school's ability to attract prospective donors and allies, and to advance the message of academic nursing practice. Moreover, these leaders are important in negotiating supportive governmental and organizational policies for the practices. An insurance executive, a physician in a large managed care insurance company, a partner in a large financial firm, an attorney, and an entrepreneur owner of a successful healthcare corporation are examples of the kind of volunteer experts appointed to the FOGP.

Through direct experience, overseers who serve on the FOGP learn much about establishing and operating clinical practices within a university context. They also learn how essential the resultant synergy among practice, research, and education is to the vibrancy and success of the school. They enjoy the contact with a very accomplished faculty and staff and increase their understanding of the professional practice of nursing. As a member of the university's trustees, the overseer chair recognizes that academic practices are an important manifestation of the university's strategic plan and goals: they provide services to the university community, are an opportunity for a trustee to make clear what the university really does and represent a logical relationship with other university resources, including its schools, departments, and health system. UPSON's overseer chair agreed to serve on the FOGP because she considered the school's vision of academic practice to be exciting and innovative, because that vision is central to the university's and the school's missions, because it illustrates the integration of the school's three components (education, research, and practice), and because it appropriately engages board members.

Overseer members of the FOGP often respond enthusiastically when asked to speak formally on academic practices from their point of view. In Tables 6.1 and 6.2, it becomes apparent from points made to audiences of other university schools of nursing from around the country just how influential the overseer's role as advisor, advocate, and ambassador is for articulating the goals of academic practices, revealing their realities, and disclosing lessons learned.

BUILDING LINKAGES FOR SUCCESS AND SUSTAINABILITY

Building a team of advisors and supporters is integral to and dovetails with ongoing development efforts. Raising funds and cultivating friends are

TABLE 6.1   Realities of Creating Academic Nursing Practices—An Overseer's View

- *No historical model.* Because the concept of school of nursing wholly-owned-and-operated nursing practices is a recent innovation, there are few historical records and lessons learned to guide designs and decisions.
- *No practical training.* Because few schools had historically assumed full responsibility for practices, there was little opportunity for deans and faculty to receive practical training in how to run such practices within a research-intensive school of nursing. In most schools, the expertise of administration, faculty, and staff has been focused on academic education and research programs.
- *Little tolerance (capital) for financial mistakes.* Schools of nursing do not have cash reserves or capital to cover mistakes or shortfalls. Therefore, there can be little tolerance within the school and the university for errors in judgment.
- *Roadblocks galore.* There are roadblocks not only on every corner, but also in the middle of the street. These roadblocks come in the form of challenges to practice privileges, HMO and individual reimbursement, physician collaboration, and marketplace competition, to name a few.
- *Lack of systems and data.* Financial and administrative systems to support billing and operations are usually nonexistent in schools of nursing. Clinical information systems need to identify the services/care provided as well as the health professional provider. Developing systems to capture each element of data to be collected requires time and resources, especially for use by nurses in primary care. Chapter 8 offers more insights into the concern for a cost-effective clinical information system (CIS).
- *Expectations of faculty.* Faculty units of measurement usually are found in teaching and scholarship, where faculty workloads are already high. Adding a practice component requires realistic balancing of faculty workload in order to accommodate practice opportunities. Some of the stresses are discussed in chapter 3.
- *Faculty and staff strengths.* Clinical knowledge, clinical skills, teaching skills, documentation skills, love of practice, and respect in the community—areas of amazing strength, creativity, and achievement—are found in the faculty and staff of schools of nursing. The challenge is to combine this exquisite capacity with business entrepreneurship to design and implement care systems that will benefit target populations.
- *Faculty and staff business acumen.* Management skills, understanding of third-party reimbursement, marketing skills, and accounting and forecasting skills are areas of expertise not usually found in faculties and staffs of schools of nursing. These are, however, the areas in which volunteer strengths can be most complementary, especially in the realm of practice. Deans, faculty, and staff need to tap volunteers with those skills. "We are delighted to volunteer where we know our skills are needed" is the response frequently heard.

TABLE 6.2   Lessons Learned—An Overseer's View

- *During early sessions, educate all parties to the same "song sheets."* Give significant time to have important discussions so that volunteers, administrators, faculty and staff can have a common understanding of the goals and accomplishments.
- *Isolate trouble spots.* Do not hesitate to identify the trouble spots with the advisory group and implement a strategy session to solve the problem as soon as possible.
- *Collectively brainstorm solutions.* Bring a broad range of expertise together to advise on the problem. For example, solving a problem of insufficient patient enrollment may require staff and volunteer expertise from marketing, clinical practice, administration, and government relations.
- *Shift thinking from practice performance to business and strategy.* It is more comfortable for nursing faculty to think about quality performance than to think about the business strategies necessary to assure the care.
- *Perform a detailed financial analysis up front to avoid surprises.* Regular/routine analyses by the staff and volunteers will identify problems in a timely fashion, at a point at which an intervention is possible. The annual report is far too late! The Financial Oversight Group for Practice reviewed detailed reports monthly.
- *Reduce every revenue expectation by 50%.* Underestimating financial projections is essential for groups that have little capital or risk reserves. Financial problems occur when projected income is spent before it accrues.
- *Manage the sales function well; reframe as "advocacy" for better faculty and staff acceptance.* Nursing faculty may not find it comfortable to be in marketing or selling.
- *Do not give full-time jobs to part-timers.* This is a frequently used operation to hold costs down; it also keeps the program from meeting its goals, however, thus creating a downward spiral.
- *Do not assume effort is the field of dreams.* "Build it and they will come" does not work well.
- *Pay attention to detail, especially expenses and accounts receivable.* An understandable finance system and reporting that is kept up daily is essential. Timely receivables are integral to an acceptable cash flow.
- *Decide on business drivers.* Identify need, competency, and payment mechanisms of the practice, then identify the key influential drivers and how to measure and monitor them regularly.
- *Report on activity versus goals.* While goals are important, tracking results of specific activities is, in reality, more helpful in determining what does and does not work.
- *Take time to reflect on, document, and disseminate lessons learned.* Faculty are better known to take time to reflect as part of scholarly activity. Engaging the volunteer advisors in this reflection is meaningful to the faculty/practitioners as well as to the volunteer. One overseer commented that the reflection that occurred with faculty and staff was something he rarely enjoyed in business.

essential to academic nursing practice sustainability. Financial support can come from individual donors (alumni, parents, family, friends), and philanthropic foundations. All are important. Donors' contributions and the very process of securing donations play critical roles in planning and successfully launching a portfolio of school-owned practices. The process of reaching out to, educating, and working with donors helps build the logic behind these practices and the stature of the practice leadership. Making the case for academic nursing practice offers another opportunity to engage more fully not only the board of overseers, but also key volunteer and philanthropic leadership and alumni, in a school's mission and programs.

The University of Pennsylvania integrates discussion of practice into all donor and community information. In addition to the creation of the FOGP, the school regularly makes the case for academic nursing practice in its own overseer board meetings through presentations on the findings of and opportunities for practice research, for clinical education, and tours of practice sites. Testimonials from patients and students are essential messages to potential donors. "Making the case" must be a top priority for administrators and faculty, as well as for the academic nursing practice staff. Advisors and supporters want to hear that the practices are part of the university and school's essential mission and that the university is supportive. They want to hear consistent messages about services and the needs those services meet. Requests for information about how things function—especially the financial support—must also be consistent. Clear, specific answers and timely responses to questions generate understanding, confidence, or enthusiasm. Sometimes this is a challenge when multiple sources of funds are necessary to keep a practice operating. Timely, clear, and accurate reports are also necessary for potential donors to understand how their contribution will "fit." UPSON is fortunate in that its Office of Development and Alumni Relations staffs the board of overseers, thus providing a strong, close linkage for all the functions and goals discussed here.

All volunteers, whether overseers, advisors, or donors, like to be taken to a practice site by the persons involved in the work and at a time when the practice is active, not when they can merely tour buildings and view empty rooms. They like to hear and experience the vision and the passion through descriptions or stories by clients or patients. The message becomes much clearer when they "visit" with nurses and patients in an active setting. These visits, although time-consuming, make academic nursing practice come alive and ultimately result in more willingness to give the much needed time and resources.

Educating those closest to the school about the importance of the practice mission and the academic practices to the school and community should lead to conversations about potential sources of funding, connections to board and alumni, and ways to present support of practice opportunities to potential donors. Prospects might be professional foundations with traditional request-for-proposal and grant application processes. For PNN, however, most potential donors were contacts made through the board or for whom a board member's endorsement proved central to cultivation.

In the process of "selling" the board on academic nursing practice, many of the hard questions for which potential supporters will want answers are identified. If the goal is raising money for school-owned academic practices, then what is the relationship of practice to the school's overall mission? How will the school balance the academic practice objectives with education and research, the other mission goals? How will the fundraising goals for academic practice fit within the university's strategic plans? The answers to these and other questions provide the basis for ongoing education aimed at internal and external constituencies.

The goal is to show—in picture and in person—what academic nursing practice looks and feels like to patients. Everyone can relate to those images of nursing, even those whose notions of the nursing profession may be more conventional and sometimes stereotypic. Often this personal connection proves more compelling to donors than simply making a fiscal case.

Making Friends and Raising Funds for Practice

Donors give money to good organizations managed by intelligent, financially astute people whose work enhances the donors' sense that they are making a positive contribution to the world. At its core, four concepts—integrity, relationships, major gifts, and reputation—should underpin a school's efforts to build strong, productive relations with donors. These concepts should be integrated into the creation and operation of key decisions, each of which should be weighed against what impact it will have on potential donors, whether that idea will present opportunities to generate and sustain revenue (donations) and, most important, how it will provide a platform to influence key decision makers. For example,

- How will a particular decision impact the promises made to donors?
- Will it improve or hurt key associations?

- What might be done to build relations further as an outcome of that decision?
- Will the decision provide an opportunity to ask someone for a major gift?
- How might the choice affect the school's reputation—with each constituency?
- What are the financial implications?
- Who else in the community endorses (and/or has already helped support) the project?

Raising money from individuals (nationwide, currently estimated to provide over 90% of all philanthropic dollars annually), corporations, and foundations is dependent on a school's ability to describe academic nursing practice as responding to real needs, having real partners, and developing realistic strategies for the future. In responding to real needs, both community and institutional, it is better to listen to the communities themselves describe their particular needs or rely on reputable source documents than for the school itself to identify those needs. Real partners are those who have experience in the field or with the practice clientele and/or have helped develop the practice itself. Developing strategies for the future means identifying what must be done when grant money runs out, and what ready-made decision and communication points exist to evaluate the progress of the practice and share that information with the donors. Prospects will ask good questions, hard questions, ones that cut to the heart of the practice initiatives, and ones that school administrators may not necessarily have asked when planning presentations and solicitations. These questions provide important opportunities to clarify key points and strategies. These questions should help shape future planning and presentations.

An important point to be made here is that the dean, faculty, and staff understand the important data that underpin the business and financial plans of the school-owned practices. Because of the complexity of practices, every effort must be made to have clear messages and descriptions. Of necessity, project goals and outcomes change frequently to keep pace with the ever-changing health care market. As these plans change, so too must the message given to volunteer leadership and donors.

In addition to government agencies, Penn Nursing secured funding for its PNN practices from a variety of sources, including professional foundations and small family foundations (see Table 6.3). In general, personal relationships made the difference in whether or not the gift or

TABLE 6.3   A Decade of Support for the Penn Nursing Network

Governmental and Philanthropic Support
for Penn Nursing Network Programs & Operations

Aetna Foundation
Allen Hilles Fund
CIGNA Foundation
City of Philadelphia Department of Health
Connelly Foundation
Danellie Foundation
Esther Gowen Hood Trust
First Hospital Foundation
Health Resources and Services Administration, Division of Nursing
Independence Foundation
Jessie Ball duPont Fund
Johnson & Johnson
Josiah Macy Jr. Foundation
Ladies Aid Society of the Presbyterian Medical Center
Patricia Kind Family Foundation
Pew Charitable Trusts
Philadelphia Health Care Trust
Presbyterian Foundation for Philadelphia
Ralston House
Robert Wood Johnson Foundation
Scholler Foundation
van Ameringen Foundation
Walter H.D. Killough Trust
William Penn Foundation
W.K. Kellogg Foundation

Research support for studies related to the Penn Nursing Network

Andrus Foundation
National Institute on Aging
National Institute for Nursing Research
Presbyterian Foundation for Philadelphia
Sigma Theta Tau
University Research Foundation

grant was secured. Traditional sources were also approached: large community and national foundations, as well as alumni, parents, faculty and friends who had the potential to make major contributions. The school talked about nursing practice and its importance everywhere and to everyone.

The strategy for fundraising also incorporated the circles of influence created by the school's volunteer leadership. An evaluation included considering whether the focus should be on major donors (gifts of $50,000 or more) or smaller ones (e.g., starting a Friends of Practice), and whether to search for new prospects or ask the school's long-standing reliable donors. Ultimately, the school chose a strategy of asking major donors who were weighted 60:30, new to old donors.

Seeking new donors offers key benefits. For example, the school's potential donor constituency was expanded by the opportunities provided to support PNN practices. Some new donors became motivated to support the school-owned practices because they can see direct effects of nurses on patient care, in contrast to support already given for scholarships and research, for example. As a result, the appeal of the academic nursing practices to new donors within the institution's overall plan grew. Also, the sphere of influence for the practice agenda in general was broadened. Among the downsides of emphasizing new donors in the development strategy are that it takes more time and effort to cultivate them, and, if they are key institutional or community donors, any failures are potentially more visible within the school's development program.

Asking for the support of longstanding school donors has benefits and challenges, too. Here, one has the opportunity to deepen and transform existing relations between the donor and school, to demonstrate to the institution the depth of the school's commitment to the specific practice and to shorten the wait for the gift. Risks may include shifting support for traditional priorities such as the annual fund or endowment to a more temporal project and, if the practice fails, risking the donor's trust and future gifts. The University of Pennsylvania's strategy was to start with new major donor prospects and ask core supporters second. Over a period of years, money was solicited and raised from foundations (local and national), individuals (board, faculty, alumni), and corporations. Each built on the other. Faculty and board giving demonstrated internal commitment. Foundation funding provided a level of security that reassured corporations.

Once the donor research is completed, the personal connections strategy identified, the proposal written, and the grant or gift secured, a stewardship plan is needed. The school and donor should identify formally or informally what the donors want in return for their support. Some formal reporting system to document outcomes heads the list. In some cases, donors want recognition through naming a space or component of the program.

Promise only what there is a reasonable chance to deliver. *It is easy to promise too much;* self sufficiency, quick operationalization, or high volume of patients are examples. It is important to identify what deliverables are actually possible, and what producing them will entail, before the gift or grant is accepted.

Delivery and infrastructure for reporting must be calculated and planned. This is critical. Future gifts can depend on one's ability to keep promises and provide accurate, timely, and thoughtful reports on the accomplishments and failures of the practice funded. Often, in the flurry of providing services, sharing timely information as a part of stewardship can be ignored.

Time is perhaps the greatest resource that will have to be calculated into garnering support for the academic practice endeavor. It is one of the most important ingredients and the one most often omitted. Educating donors about the value and reality of academic nursing practices takes time and repetition. Working with volunteers and donors is usually not efficient, simple, or systematic. Be ready when they are. Volunteer leadership and donors require individual attention—to their concerns, questions, needs, and timelines. It takes time to communicate to and with everyone, to follow through and answer all questions. It means operating on donors' timetables, not the school's, using their language, not nursing's—especially not jargon or acronyms familiar only to nurses and health professionals. Donors and volunteers usually have their primary focus on other important matters. It takes time to think of ways to involve them and to keep them involved, focused, and informed about the positive outcomes of academic nursing practice. It takes time to share with them the words and feelings of patients and the community—not in a photocopied narrative, but one-on-one. One of nursing's best selling points is that nurses *do spend time* with patients. This same investment will ensure the health of fundraising for practices. It is also a key feature in producing a successful communications strategy.

PROMOTING THE MESSAGE

In addition to informing the volunteer leadership, advisors and financial supporters, academic nursing practice has important messages to share with the public, with patients, with policy makers, and with professional colleagues. This can be accomplished through three marketing mainstays: advertising, special events, and publicity. Advertising is the promotional and informational literature and paid advertisements that allow a school to say what it wants to say when it wants to say them. Special events introduce a targeted group or groups to a particular academic practice by bringing them to the facility, generally by means of some combination of a ribbon-cutting ceremony, open house, and/or health fair. While such community-based special events may generate publicity in the form of a daily newspaper article or local news broadcast, they should not be planned with that as a primary goal. There are no guarantees that the media will consider the event newsworthy. Alternatively, publicity is the dissemination of news and information through the print, broadcast, and electronic media. Not only is publicity difficult to control, but the organization, whether school or academic nursing practice, has no control over the final story. A clear advantage is that the publicity is free and, when it succeeds, can yield exponential returns across a broad audience.

In the early stages of planning, the development of the school-owned practices (i.e., PNN), the counsel of a well-respected local marketing firm that specialized in health care helped to clarify marketing goals and objectives and confirmed what the school had already determined as its target audiences. The firm developed a logo (corporate identity) for PNN and recommended a series of advertising and direct mail campaigns. Those campaigns, while ideal, were well outside the school's budget. Advertising was streamlined to capitalize on existing communications and media relations resources within the school and the university. In-house writing talent and desktop publishing were used for PNN brochures and a limited number of targeted advertisements were placed. A restricted budget, however, need not unduly constrain marketing efforts. Through careful, well-conceived planning and the leveraging of existing expertise, PNN achieved effective publicity in local newspapers, on television and radio, and in periodicals aimed at health care providers.

That planning consisted of identifying the audience, the message, and the "hook." Particularly important in promoting the PNN were eight key audiences:

1. Health care professionals, whose referrals were needed.
2. Insurers, whose reimbursement was essential.
3. The community—an important source of patients and good will.
4. Legislators and government officials, whose understanding of and legislative support critical issues, such as advanced practice nurses,

reimbursement for those nurses, and funding education, was important.

5. University officials, whose backing to the success of PNN at many levels was crucial.

6. Funders, whose support, particularly at the start-up stages, was pivotal.

7. Prospective students, who could see a tangible tripartite learning model firsthand.

8. Academic nursing, to whom UPSON could advance its reputation as a leader.

Once the audiences are identified, a targeted message can be shaped to each constituency using the best possible methods. For example, telling the community about the University of Pennsylvania's academic nursing practices meant helping the public understand what nurse practitioners were and what qualified them to provide basic health care services competently. The best way to tell that story—again, on a shoestring budget—is through strategically placed articles in weekly community newspapers that will be read by the same public that PNN practices would serve (e.g., Asthma education, 1998; Glancaterino, 1998; Swan, 1998). To influence colleagues in health care to refer patients to those practices, stories need to be placed in professional publications that those providers would read. The message to those colleagues often focused on research findings that supported the role of advanced practice nurses as providers of primary care (e.g., Evans, Yurkow, & Siegler, 1995; Lang & Evans, 1999; Naylor & Buhler-Wilkerson, 1999). Funders and legislators learn the public value of Penn's nursing practices through newspaper articles in major dailies that focused on how Penn's academic nursing practices increase access to basic health services (e.g., Russ, 1995; McCollum, 1995).

Finding the "Hook"

Once the individual messages to targeted audiences are shaped, the question becomes how to influence a journalist that the desired message is interesting and newsworthy and that the story should be told. This requires a good hook, one that may be as simple as, "Our town has never had a midwifery practice." Or, in the case of PNN's Health Annex, "to house our practice, we renovated a deteriorating community recreation center."

The challenge of placing a story and developing a strong hook varies, depending on the intended medium and geographic region or area of the practice(s). Major dailies in large cities, where competition for stories is high, for example, can be harder to penetrate than a weekly community paper looking for personal interest stories of immediate neighborhood interest. The same can be said for placing a TV news story in a major city, where competing for the attention of a news editor or producer is far more difficult than it would be in a smaller town.

Lessons in Building Media Relations

Using the media to help promote academic nursing practice can be one of the most effective marketing tools. Not every effort will succeed, however, and faculty and staff must be counted on to spend countless hours talking with reporters and editors to help launch and sustain efforts. The University of Pennsylvania's most valuable lessons in how to build a successful media relations program can be distilled into five principles: educate, educate, and educate again; humanize the story; look beyond the obvious; think fast; and, as with advisor and donor relations, be prepared to invest time.

Educate, Educate, and Educate Again. Educate reporters not once but continually. Most reporters have little understanding of what advanced practice nurses are, much less what their educational requirements are, the scope of their practice, and that they are highly skilled professionals able to practice independently. When talking with a reporter about a school's academic nursing practices, invite the person to visit the site to interview staff and patients and provide detailed background about the program(s) in question and the kinds and number of patients cared for, as well as any honors or awards received. Equally important is to inform the reporter about advanced practice nurses (APNs), the particular distinctiveness of the school's graduate programs, and the research and data that support the role of APNs.

An example is helpful to understanding how these multiple messages are included. When Penn Nursing pitched the opening of its Living Independently For Elders (LIFE) to the *Philadelphia Business Journal*, the region's largest, most influential business weekly, the paper's health care reporter was invited to the practice site. While interviewing faculty co-directors, the reporter learned not just about LIFE, but about all the other Penn Nursing Network practices as well. He left with detailed information about numbers of patients served, awards received, and research supporting the importance of nurse practitioners. Several days later, the reporter called with information about the paper's annual Healthcare Heroes Award, which recognized organizations and people in the Philadelphia region who had made a significant contribution to the health and well-being of area residents. He suggested that PNN enter the competition. Several weeks later, it was learned that PNN had received honorable mention. Part of that award included an article in the Healthcare Heroes supplement of the *Philadelphia Business Journal* (George, 1998). Later, the reporter told us how impressed he had been, not only with LIFE, but also with all the other practices. Until his interview, he said, he had had no idea what a nurse practitioner does.

Humanize the Story. Humanizing the story is one of the easiest things that nursing can do. At its core, nursing is about caring for people. Human-interest stories naturally abound from the relationship between nursing and the patient. One of the best ways to explain the value of nursing care and APNs is to have patients tell the story by sharing their experience.

For example, when the University of Pennsylvania developed the press release for The Collaborative Assessment and Rehabilitation for Elders (CARE) Program (see Exemplar), instead of trying to describe the rather complex practice concept to a lay audience, a case study of Mrs. X was created to explain the benefits of The CARE Program to patients and their families. A patient was identified who was willing to talk with reporters about his experience with the program. In many ways, such human interest stories can portray the unique partnership among "people" from the respective school, the practice and the community in which it is based, and the city or the region.

Look beyond the obvious. Looking beyond the obvious is what to do when, despite all the pitching and talking and educating, reporters cannot be convinced that the story is worth telling. So, when all else fails, try another angle, and broaden the outreach beyond the health care reporter.

A journalist who covered Philadelphia neighborhoods for the region's largest daily newspaper was moved by the remarks of the city's recreation commissioner, who spoke of the remarkable crew of city workmen who used their craft and skill to restore a decaying recreation center in one of the city's most neglected high-crime areas, then the future site of the PNN Health Annex. Pitching the Health Annex as a neighborhood story, the investment of the school, the city, and the neighbors in restoring the recreation center had been emphasized. But there in plain view were the workmen. Who would have imagined that plumbers and carpenters would have been the linchpin for a cover story published in the Sunday magazine section of the paper, one written not by a health reporter but by a person who specializes in writing about Philadelphia's neighborhoods (Kadaba, 1996).

Think Fast. Thinking fast in media relations parlance is simply staying nimble enough to roll with the punches, whether those issues concern turning problems into opportunities or larger news stories for which your particular expertise can be important. The closure of The CARE Program presented an interesting dilemma. Should a press release be issued proactively about the program's closure (see Chapter 4), using the story to tell the public about how changes in Medicare reimbursement policy affected services for rehabilitation for frail older people? Or, given the prevailing politics, was staying under the radar more advisable so as not to draw attention to a failure for nursing practices? One of the city's councilwomen was a strong supporter of the University of Pennsylvania. Because her mother had benefited from the services of The CARE Program, the councilwoman encouraged getting the word out, and she offered to be a spokesperson for the program. In the process of deciding strategy, Penn developed a list of talking points for The CARE Program director in the event a reporter contacted her about the program's closing. Several weeks later, a *Wall Street Journal* article appeared about the capping of payments to nursing homes for rehabilitation services. Those talking points were immediately turned into a letter to the editor in which Penn's experience with such cuts (70% to be exact) in reimbursement to free-standing outpatient rehabilitation services was described—cuts that forced the closure of The CARE Program. When that letter was published (Lang, 1999), copies were sent to colleagues throughout the university, including the president and provost, as well as to state and federal senators and members of congress and to those of their staff involved in setting Medicare policy.

Be Prepared to Invest Time. Finally, media relations, like development, is an investment in time. Persistence is key in working with the media. Some stories make it. Others do not. Still others become stories months or years after they are first presented to the media. Such was the case with the Health Annex at the Francis J. Myers Recreation Center. Four years after trying to pitch the story to local television news stations, a producer at the city's most popular station called us based on that four-year-old press release. She was interested in doing a story on physicians' assistants and nurse practitioners as professionals who were replacing physicians and who had a fairly controversial bias. Penn immediately sent her lots of information about the Health Annex, numbers of patients served, health promotion programs offered, and research supporting nurse practitioners. She was impressed and wanted to recast her story in a more positive light.

With a camera crew, she came to the Health Annex. In advance, PNN arranged to have available for interviews a family who had received all their primary care there. The director and a nurse practitioner spent hours preparing for their interviews, and another several hours waiting to be interviewed. That effort, which had begun some four years ago, paid off with a local news story that ran on both the 6:00 p.m. and 11:00 p.m. broadcasts.

Inherent in all these strategies is one overriding message: If good working relations are developed with the media, those journalists can be among a school's greatest allies in advancing nursing practices. Achieving and sustaining that rapport means respecting reporters' deadlines, responding immediately to their requests for information and interviews, not wasting their time with stories that have no news value, and becoming dependable news sources by being well-prepared for each interview with a list of no more than three talking points. In the end, adopting these core principles is one of the best antidotes to the persistently common misperception among many nurses that "medicine makes headlines, nursing does not."

BLUEPRINT FOR SUCCESS

By including school-owned practices within an academic nursing practice portfolio, schools of nursing face a number of challenges. Asking for the right help is an effective way to meet those challenges. In choosing to establish an advisory group, such as a financial oversight committee, the school (specifically the dean and director of the academic practices) secures a powerful resource through which to understand the realities of academic practice, how to handle such challenges as achieving financial health, being entrepreneurs as well as academicians, finding the best fit in the health care delivery system, securing university support and buy-in, and understanding "when to hold and when to fold."

Clearly, the advisory group can also help develop a blueprint for success and, by definition, minimize risk. One FOGP member at Penn Nursing explained that blueprint this way: "To succeed, take advantage of experts. Be flexible enough to adapt to market trends. Learn more about marketing, planning, development and communication. Develop good business skills, but do not wait for the perfect model to get started. Instead, realize that several stages of development and evolution will be inevitable. Understand the environment and adapt to it. Secure and expand buy-in from as many constituents as possible who will be affected, and develop staying power to weather the storms" (Overseers & Advisors, 1999, 2000). From Penn

Nursing's perspective, the road to that success can be possible by gathering the right people, asking the right questions, and re-asking better questions. Equally important is to admit it when wrong, learn from mistakes, minimize losses, and respond rapidly. Above all, celebrate successes and hold on to the passions that brought everyone to the table in the first place.

ACKNOWLEDGMENTS

In addition to the Honorable Marjorie O. Rendell, Jeffrey Levitt, Catherine R. Judge and Susan Greenbaum, the contributions of Vivian Piasecki, Joseph Carver, Steven Golding, Kathleen Welsh Beveridge, Catherine Dougherty Greenland, Mary Burke, Dennis Matthews, Patrick Burke and Joy McIntyre are gratefully acknowledged. Without their wise counsel and assistance at every turn, the vision would not have taken flight, much less been realized.

Exemplar A.
The Collaborative Assessment and Rehabilitation for Elders (CARE) Program.

As Penn Nursing began to inform the media about its new practice, The CARE Program, colleagues in health care who were important referral sources for the practice were identified as the primary audience. Because of the important role of advanced practice nurses in providing quality, cost-effective care to a most vulnerable population, namely, frail elders, a wider audience was targeted: university officials, the community, legislators, funders, insurers, and others. A message began to be shaped that would attract both the health care and the general media; namely, that based on years of research and experience in caring for older patients, the University of Pennsylvania School of Nursing (UPSON) had a way to improve function and quality of life for frail elders.

Part of the first public message involved a ribbon-cutting ceremony—a special event—that would draw the target audiences to the facility. Although press coverage was not the top priority in planning this event, television coverage for our opening did occur, probably, because several important government officials were part of the ceremony. In addition, the program's director appeared on several public affairs TV shows aimed at an elderly population. In the Philadelphia market, these shows tend to air very early in the morning, attracting large numbers of viewers who watch because of what experts have to say about issues relevant to aging.

Delivering the full message about The CARE Program in a press release to be distributed to health care print and broadcast journalists was challenging. Because the message of CARE was a complicated one for a lay audience, a clear, compelling story with a strong hook was needed. Drawing on health care reform debate from the early 1990s, then often in the news, the message was shaped around The CARE Program as an innovative solution to the nation's health care crisis, particularly as it related to our elderly population. The press release headline read, "On the Leading Edge of Health Care Reform," and the text used such buzzwords as "cost-effective," "high quality," and "alternative to nursing-home placement." A corresponding fact sheet answered specific questions about CARE. Because The CARE Program's concept was complex, the story was told through the eyes of patients who would benefit from the program.

To reach the primary audience—health care providers and insurers—the press release was sent to Philadelphia area health care publications that feature regional news and trends. That resulted in articles in several periodicals (News in Brief, 1994; Nurse-managed Day hospital, 1995; Yurkow & Greenbaum, 1995).

Over the years, UPSON continued to receive coverage of The CARE Program's story in national nursing and health care publications on the basis of articles submitted by UPSON staff and faculty (Evans, Yurkow, & Siegler, 1994; Evans, Yurkow, & Siegler, 1995; Naylor & Buhler-Wilkerson, 1999; Reed, 1997). This effort was an important factor in establishing the University of Pennsylvania as a leader in academic nursing practice.

—Susan Greenbaum

REFERENCES

Evans, L., Yurkow, J., & Siegler, E. (1994). A nurse-managed collaborative outpatient program to improve function in the frail elderly [Abstract]. *Gerontologist, 34* (Special Issue 1), 265.

Evans, L. K., Yurkow, J., & Siegler, E. L. (1995). The CARE Program: A nurse-managed collaborative outpatient program to improve function of frail older people. *Journal of the American Geriatric Society, 43,* 1155–1160.

George, J. (October 26, 1998). Focus: Health care heroes. Penn Nursing: Providing primary care. *Philadelphia Business Journal*, 8–9.

Kadaba, L. S. (January 21, 1996). Work of heart: From wrecked center to rec center, with love. *Philadelphia Inquirer Sunday Magazine*, 7.

Lang, N. M. (May 13, 1999). Letters to the Editor. Medicare provisions in '97 Act are flawed. *The Wall Street Journal*.

Lang, N. M., & Evans, L. (1999). Case study: Forging new partnerships for financial development: The experience of the Penn Nursing Network. In J. A. Ryan (Ed.), *Managing market demand for nursing services: The nurse executive role* (pp. 115–124). Chicago: AONE/Health Forum.

Naylor, M. D., & Buhler-Wilkerson, K. (1999). Creating community-based care for the new millennium. *Nursing Outlook, 47*(3), 120–127.

News in brief (1994, February 28–March 13). Penn Nursing School initiates outpatient program for elderly. *Nurse Extra, 5*.

Nurse-managed day hospital stresses independent living. (January, 1995). *Hospital News/Philadelphia*, 9.

Overseers and Advisors (July 1999,July 2000). *Why academic nursing practice? The business of practice—Finding expertise*. Panel presentation to Penn Macy Institute. Philadelphia: University of Pennsylvania School of Nursing.

Reed, D. (1997). Development of a community-based, nurse-managed practice network by the University of Pennsylvania School of Nursing. In *The third national primary care conference: Case studies in community-based academic partnerships* (pp. 129–140). Washington, DC: Health Resources & Services Administration.

Yurkow, J., & Greenbaum, S. (1995). C.A.R.E. for the elderly makes a difference. *NPNews, 5*(4).

Chapter 7

Infrastructure to Support Academic Nursing Practice[1]

Beth Ann Swan

Exemplars by Betty S. Adler, Melinda Jenkins, and Eileen Sullivan-Marx

With the rapid expansion of academic nursing practice portfolios of U.S. schools of nursing to include equity practices, recognition is growing that adoption of a sound set of business principles is essential if these initiatives are to be established, nurtured, and sustained. The success and failure of many academic practices has rested on the degree to which a school of nursing (SON) has been able to embrace and integrate business principles to guide its practice initiatives (Vincent, Oakley, Pohl, & Walker, 2000). A range of business principles, models, and organizational structures (Barnett, Niebuhr, & Baldwin, 1998; Foxcroft, Cole, Fulbrook, Johnston, & Stevens, 2001; Friedman et al., 1999; Guarino, 1997; Hardy, 2000; Hill, 2001; Hoffman et al., 1995; Neumann, Blouin, & Byrne, 1999; Pardes, 1997; Smith & Bryant, 1988; West, 2002)

---

[1]Portions of this chapter are reprinted from *Nursing Economic$*, 2001, Volume 19, Number 2, pp. 68–71, by permission of the publisher (Jannetti Publications, East Holly Avenue Box 56, Pitman, NJ 08071-0056).

are applicable to schools planning to develop, finance, and evaluate an academic practice. These principles are useful regardless of the type(s) of practice(s) offered, which may include primary or long-term care, interdisciplinary health care, health promotion and prevention services (see also Chapters 3 & 4). Following a brief discussion of business concepts and organizational structure, a case study of the University of Pennsylvania School of Nursing's (UPSON) Penn Nursing Network (PNN) is used to exemplify an organizing framework for planning infrastructure essential to sustaining an academic practice. Exemplars are included that depict critical legal and risk management principles and the importance of addressing potential state and federal regulatory barriers to the conduct of academic nursing practice.

BUSINESS CONCEPTS AND ORGANIZATIONAL STRUCTURE

Business concept innovation is the capacity to imagine dramatically different business concepts or dramatically new ways of differentiating existing business concepts. The goal of business concept innovation is to introduce more strategic variety into an industry, in this case into academic nursing practice (Christensen, 2000; Eisenhardt & Brown, 1999; Evans & Wurster, 2000; Hagel & Singer, 1999; Hamel, 2000; Moore, 2000). The components of a business model include core strategy, customer interface, strategic resources, and value network. *Core strategy* is the fundamental nature of how a practice or business chooses to compete. Elements of the core strategy include the mission, service scope, and basis for differentiation (how the practice competes differently from its competitors; Hamel, 2000). *Customer interface* includes four essentials: fulfillment and support, information and insight, relationship dynamics, and pricing structure. Fulfillment and support refers to the way the practice reaches clients and patients and the level of service that is provided. Information and insight encompasses all the knowledge that is collected from and utilized on behalf of clients and patients to develop and implement creative services for them. Relationship dynamics refers to the nature of the interaction between providers and clients, from face-to-face to virtual. Pricing structure is the financial arrangements between providers, patients, and payers, whether patients pay fee for service or through some third-party arrangement (Hagel & Singer, 1999). *Strategic resources* include core competencies, core processes, and strategic assets. The skills and unique structural capabilities of a practice represent its core competencies, whereas core processes are the activities themselves. Strategic assets include infrastructure, technology, data, and anything else that is unique and valuable. The fourth component of a business model is the *value network* that surrounds the practice and complements and augments the practice's own resources (Hamel, 2000). Partners and collaborators form this network.

Unfortunately, organizational structures rarely result from systematic, methodical planning. Rather, they evolve over time, "in fits and starts, shaped more by politics than by policies" (Goold & Campbell, 2000, p. 117). The chaotic nature of the resulting structure is, then, more often a function of crisis management and a source of constant frustration for practice leadership and staff. Strategic initiatives stall or go astray because responsibilities may be unclear or disjointed. Turf wars bring to a standstill collaboration and knowledge sharing. Promising opportunities die for lack of attention and ownership of the initiative. Organizational structures become inefficient because of lack of clarity about responsibilities. Given this typical haphazard development, a business model that begins with an assessment of organizational structures including core strategy, customer interface, strategic resources, and value network is a logical first step when planning any new business/practice venture (Buppert, 1999).

ACADEMIC NURSING PRACTICE AS A BUSINESS

Academic nursing practices—in which schools of nursing deliberately integrate research, education, and clinical services—provide models of cost-effective care to multiple client populations across the care continuum. As described in Chapter 4, schools of nursing have historically confined their foci to teaching and research and consequently have had little experience with conducting the business of health care. Further, neither traditional organizational structures nor systems for finance and business, legal, risk management, information, marketing, and so on translate well to the business of practice. This is certainly underscored in the experience of UPSON, which, in 1994, established PNN as part of its strategic plan to more fully operationalize its integrated tripartite mission (Evans, Jenkins, & Buhler-Wilkinson, 2003). PNN has operated simultaneously up to 10 small and dissimilar practices providing primary care and specialty services to women and children, families, adults, frail elders, and providers. Since inception of PNN, the school has required many financial and nonfinancial resources to mount, build, and sustain such an ambitious undertaking (Lang & Evans,

1999). One of the essential ingredients for success was an infrastructure for practice.

The *American Heritage Dictionary of the English Language* (1996) defines infrastructure as "an underlying base or foundation especially for an organization or a system; the basic facilities, services, and installations needed for the functioning of a community" (p. 927). Infrastructure for the educational and research components of the tripartite mission are well established in schools of nursing in research-intensive universities. Infrastructure in support of clinical practice, however, requires a different set of skills and functions that may not readily be molded from existing resources. Building and financially supporting such an infrastructure can be critical to the business success of the clinical practice arm. Schools of nursing in liberal arts colleges will differ from those in schools with academic medical centers in terms of the resources on which they can draw in deciding about and developing an infrastructure for practice. Financing such infrastructure will be shaped by existing policy at each institution. At a private university, such as the University of Pennsylvania, for example, it is expected that each school will "rest on its own bottom" financially. The practice venture, a substantial component of the school's operation, must do the same, with no cushion, either at the university or at the school level. The experiences of PNN are used here for illustrative purposes.

CASE STUDY: PENN NURSING NETWORK

Over its lifespan, the PNN has encompassed a broad range of practices (see Chapter 4 & Table 5.2 in Chapter 5), from primary care to nurse midwifery to capitated risk-based services for frail elders. Prior to 1994, each of UPSON's existing practices had provided for its own basic business needs, and/or existing administrative services in UPSON had been stretched to encompass the practice initiative. As PNN became more formalized, one of the first steps for the leadership was to identify the foundational services that the practices would require in order to do business. The leadership then determined methods for acquiring and paying for all these services. Consultants assisted in laying out infrastructure components (see Table 7.1) and framework for decision making (see Chapter 4 and Table 7.2). Some overarching considerations in the decision to use a combination of "make, use, and buy" strategies (Porter, 1998) included: (1) availability of existing services, including timeliness and turnaround time; (2) skills of existing internal staff and external vendors; (3) investment, operating and, liability costs; and (4) need for control.

TABLE 7.1   Practice Infrastructure Needs

Administrative Support	Insurance & Risk Management
Billing & Collections	Legal
Business Planning & New Ventures	Managed Care Relations
Communications	Marketing
Continuing Education	Media & Public Relations
Contracting & Negotiating	Policies & Procedures
Credentialing	Practice Management Oversight
Development	Purchasing
Facilities Management	Quality Management
Finance/Budgeting/Accounting	Reimbursement
Government Relations	Security
Grants Management	Strategic Planning
Human Resources	System Development & Management
Information Systems	

Infrastructure Strategies

As specified in the initial strategic plan, infrastructure to support the practice initiative is determined through strategic evaluation of resources that should be created within PNN ("make"), those that were available within UPSON and the university ("use"), and/or those that should be purchased from outside vendors ("buy"). As a strategic principle, PNN focused its own primary resources on clinical services development, service delivery, and quality management, relying on a lean infrastructure (a combination primarily of "make" and "use" services) for other support functions. When "using" services from the university, everyone had the same goal in mind—to help meet the mission in as risk-free way as possible. Sometimes this translated to a risk-management strategy that weighed the risks and benefits and resulted in a conservative approach, not necessarily unwillingness to help with SON goals. It was up to the practice leadership to educate the university departments' leadership on the benefits, to work with them to minimize risks in the processes that were set up, and to develop good partnerships and relations with these offices. Using these strategies, in 1994, a central infrastructure with staff positions was first created for PNN. The goal of the infrastructure was to provide overall direction, oversight, and support to PNN practices in order to achieve strategic objectives as defined by the faculty (Lang & Evans, 1999).

In examining infrastructure requirements for academic nursing practice, it should be noted that the majority of functions identified are similar to

TABLE 7.2 Infrastructure Options and Criteria

OPTION	DEFINITION	DECISION CRITERIA	ACTION
Make	Created within PNN and supported by PNN staff positions	– Service requires a central locus of control – Internal competencies exist	– Define service and staff requirements – Determine if and for what services PNN may wish/need to retain control – Execute "make" strategies
Use	Accessed within the school of nursing and/or university	– Service will be supportive, timely, responsive – Competencies are relevant to the practice(s) – Cost–quality trade-off is favorable	– Identify, if any, existing services within the school of nursing and/or university – Set parameters for services to use – Define contract or agreement
Buy	Contracted with external vendors	– Financial risk is negligible or within reason – Buying decreases the need for start-up capital – Buying leverages existing market skills – Buying avoids wasting energy and time – Service is definitely needed	– Identify potential vendors – Hold initial exploratory meetings with vendors – Request proposals – Review proposals and modify contract drafts – Select vendor – Negotiate details – Execute contract – Continually evaluate readiness of organization to establish in-house infrastructure services

those provided by separate departments in academic health centers, for example, finance, accounting, billing and collections, new ventures and business planning, grants management, government relations, human resources, information systems, marketing, and legal. Schools of nursing within an academic health science center/medical center may be better positioned to use services from specific departments in the health science center. UPSON, however, is autonomous from the University of Pennsylvania Medical Center or Health System, and PNN lacked the resources required to support this level of infrastructure for itself. Thus, PNN was dependent on non–health care departments to either perform or outsource the practice-related work. For example, in the mid-1990s, there existed at the University of Pennsylvania a separation between legal departments for the university and the health system. SON legal services were handled by the university legal department, which outsourced legal work for The CARE Program, a SON clinical practice, since no one in that office had expertise in the Medicare rules and regulations governing comprehensive outpatient rehabilitation facilities (CORFs). There was also a need to work with the university risk management office regarding specialized malpractice, liability insurance requirements, plan for reporting and handling occurrences, and so on. Legal principles to consider when doing academic practice are discussed in Exemplar A at the end of this chapter.

Potential resources may exist in other university offices. For example, the government relations office may be helpful in clarifying and helping achieve change in state and federal regulatory restrictions affecting full implementation of the academic practice plan; where universities and colleges do not have such resources on site, they may need to look to other sources of support, including collaborative and cooperative networks (see Chapter 12). For PNN to help demonstrate the value added by advanced practice nurse (APN) services, the practice environments needed to be reshaped and changed from a regulatory and payment perspective. PNN leadership established an association with the university's government relations office in order to update continually and seek assistance as needed on multiple federal- and state-level issues that impacted the practices (refer to Exemplars B and C).

Early on, it became apparent that continually assessing, evaluating, and "rightsizing" the infrastructure would be key for strategic planning, day-to-day operations, and survival (Swan & Evans, 2001). The budget for PNN "make" and "buy" infrastructure was derived from the indirect charges levied against each practice and from grants and gifts. PNN supported its "use" infrastructure functions through paying its share of allocated costs to UPSON and the university. Initial "make" infrastructure positions included the following: (1) director for academic nursing practice, a standing faculty member who had leadership and oversight for the academic nursing practice mission; (2) group practice administrator/chief financial officer, and (3) office administrative assistant. As the practices grew, the following positions were created: (1) billing manager, (2) billing clerk, (3) financial analyst, (4) associate director for operations in a modified chief operating officer role, (5) network operations manager, (6) information systems coordinator, (7) quality management consultant, and (8) special projects coordinator. Over the last eight years, the infrastructure has been dynamic, expanding to as high as 8.75 full-time employees (FTEs) and contracting to 2.90 FTEs to meet the changing size and needs of the practices. Some examples of the functions provided by the PNN infrastructure are illustrated in Table 7.3.

More recently, a decision was made to maintain strategic planning, monitoring, analysis, system and new service development, and quality management at the PNN infrastructure level, while functions over which the practice managers need direct control are gradually being moved to the level of the individual practice (Swan, 2000; Swan & Cotroneo, 1999). In large part, this decision was driven by the disparate needs of very different practice models within PNN. The practice-level functions include credentialing with insurers, medical assistance, Medicare, managed care; practice-specific contract negotiations and management; policies and procedures; strategic planning and marketing; facilities management, and clinical billing and collections. There are specific aspects to each of these functions.

For clinical billing and collections, recent developments and ongoing changes in reimbursement regulations and payment structures of many health care plans—Medicare, Medicaid, and commercial insurers—led PNN to evolve from an initial "make" strategy (PNN infrastructure performing this function) to a "buy" strategy (outsourcing billing and collections) and back to a "make" strategy (performing function, but at the level of individual practices). On a national level, many schools with academic practices are contemplating or beginning to use outsourcing ("buy" strategy), especially for billing and collections.

For facilities management, functions may entail space utilization and rental; interior and exterior preventive maintenance; heating, ventilation, and air conditioning (HVAC); power; electric, telephone, water; interior and exterior repairs; housekeeping; and preparing space for events, as well as preparing sites for opening, moving, and closing. In closing a practice,

TABLE 7.3   Infrastructure Function Strategies of the Penn Nursing Network Over Time

Functions	Strategy FY1999	Strategy FY2000	Strategy FY2001	Strategy FY2002

Administrative Support
  Staffing multiple commit-
    tees and meetings
  Scheduling meetings and
    appointments
  Correspondence
  Typing and maintaining
    official files
	Make	Make	Make/Use	Use

Business Planning & New
  Ventures
  Business Plan
    Consultation
  Practice Diversification
    Consultation
  Managed Care Negotia-
    tion Consultation
	Make/Buy	Make/Buy	Make/Buy	Use/Buy

Credentialing	Make	Make	Make	Make

Finance
  Accounting
  Analysis & Projections
  Banking
  Billing & Collections
  Budgeting
  Compliance with
    Federal & State
    Regulations
  Payables & Purchasing
  Report Preparation
	Make/Buy/
	Use*
		Make/Use*	Make/Use*	Use*

Grants Management	Make/Use*	Make/Use*	Make/Use*	Use*
Human Resources	Make/Use*	Make/Use*	Make/Use*	Use*
Information Systems	Make/Use*	Make/Use*	Make/Use*	Use*
Legal & Risk Management	Use*	Use*	Use*	Use*
Marketing, Media, & Public Relations	Make/Use*	Make/Use*	Make/Use*	Use*

*Functions supported by University of Pennsylvania School of Nursing and University of Pennsylvania

some of the same facilities management issues need to be addressed, including terms and payment of leases for space; completing an inventory; redistributing, storing, and/or selling furniture, equipment, and supplies; and removing signage. It is important to contact the legal department at the beginning of the process. From a legal/risk management perspective, it also is important to comply with requirements for archiving records for future access and to provide written notification to patients of their options, providers of their responsibilities and payers and anyone with whom the practice has had contracts or other business arrangements re: the practice status.

Financing Infrastructure

As mentioned previously, most of the cost for the central PNN infrastructure is supported by an indirect rate levied against each practice (currently 10% of expenditures), with the remainder supported by gifts and grants. In accordance with existing university policy, the indirect rate structure was based on a similar calculation formula used for determining UPSON's allocated costs to the university. The PNN contribution to allocated costs supports its use of UPSON services such as business, development, and public relations offices and university services such as legal, risk management, payroll, human resources, and so on. When appropriate, infrastructure support is included in grant proposals. Direct project grants have permitted PNN to bring on line more rapidly new infrastructure positions or functions than might have been possible by relying entirely on revenue from the indirect rate assessment. As painfully discovered, planning for continuing support once grant funding is ended must be part of the strategy from the start.

In FY 1999, for example, the PNN information systems infrastructure (1.4 FTEs) was supported entirely with grant funding. These staff positions provided information technology support to all the PNN practices and included basic computer hardware and software purchasing, installation, and maintenance; software purchasing, installation, training, and maintenance for various patient registration and billing software; development, installation, and training for a new point-of-service clinical information system; and 24 hours per day, seven days per week system and desktop support and troubleshooting. Planning for continuation beyond the grant period had not been fully implemented, and the PNN staff positions could no longer be supported within the existing PNN budget. Of necessity, PNN initially employed the "use" strategy and tried to depend on UPSON's information systems (IS) department to meet these needs. This approach, however, was not fully workable. While knowledgeable about the education and research environment and needs, UPSON's IS staff were not familiar with the clinical practice setting and were unequipped to travel to off-site locations for basic installations and support. Neither were they well-versed in patient registration, billing, or electronic clinical information systems, nor geared to provide 24/7 system support. Accordingly, a PNN information technology strategic plan, which included financing to place this function back into the PNN infrastructure ("make"), was developed and implemented.

The clinical academic nursing practice component of a school's mission is actually a business with its own unique and specialized infrastructure needs. Schools contemplating development or expansion of the practice mission would do well to factor into the strategic plan a range of graduated methods to provide necessary infrastructure. Underestimating the financial resources required to support these practice initiatives and the sheer inability to "add on" specialized requirements to already stressed and ill-equipped systems existing within the school is a recipe for disaster. Strategic planning (including assurance of funding support) for establishing and then sustaining ongoing operations of the infrastructure is essential to success.

Exemplar A.
Legal Principles to Consider when Doing Academic Practice.

Legal Issues

Over the lifespan of the academic practice, you will need to work with your attorney(s) in varied contexts related to:

- *Establishing the practice (setting up an academic practice is setting up a business)*
- *Setting up a governance structure*
- *Contracting for additional services or with payors*
- *Complying with Medicare and Medicaid policies and other state and federal laws*
- *Closing a practice or what to do when a provider leaves a practice*

Get to know your attorney and work with her on:

- *Regulatory Issues*
- *Transactions and Contracts*
- *Corporate Issues*
- *Governance*
- *Reimbursement*
- *Operations and Clinical Matters*

Communicate with your attorney:

- *Explain the facts*
- *Educate him about your practice needs and style.*

Allow for reasonable completion time, plus some:

- *Drafting, negotiation, and waiting for responses from the other side always take longer than you wish.*
- *Work together to achieve the right level of risk for your institution*

Licensure and Compliance

Complying with state and federal licensing and regulatory requirements is important in academic practice; maintaining compliance with requirements for scope of practice and federal and state billing and reimbursement regulations are especially critical areas.

Entity may need to fall within the state's licensing of facilities. For example, adult daycare, ambulatory surgery, long-term nursing facility. Some states may still have certificate of need programs as well.

Individual Providers

- *Scope of license for nurses and advanced practice nurses*
- *Scope of practice driven by licensure (State law) and billing (Federal and State law)*
- *Certified Registered Nurse Practitioners (CRNPs) must practice consistent with agreement with collaborating physician*
- *CRNPs must practice consistent with rules governing certain health care settings*

Anti-Kickback Prohibition

- *Referrals of Medicare and Medicaid patients. Federal anti-kickback law prohibits providers from knowingly or willfully soliciting or accepting "remuneration" directly or indirectly for referrals of Medicare or Medicaid patients; remuneration can be a payment, kickback, gift, or bribe in the form of cash, services or equipment and is intent-based.*
- *Bottom line: Cannot pay for patient referrals.*
- *Violation can result in imprisonment, civil fines, exclusion from Medicare and Medicaid programs, and loss of license.*
- *"Safe harbors" protect some business practices and relationships that would otherwise be illegal such as certain lease arrangements, personal service contracts, management agreements.*

False Claims

- *Healthcare providers are prohibited from making false statements or representations to the government in an application under Medicare or Medicaid programs. False claims can occur through billing and reimbursement; for example, billing for Advanced Practice Nurses (APNs) independently is different from billing for APNs "incident to."*

Documentation

- *"If it is not documented, it did not happen."*
- *Quality concerns*
- *Reimbursement concerns*
- *Concerns when defending a lawsuit*

Transactions and Contracts

Academic practices will contract with many parties in establishing and maintaining the practice—including, for example, providers, third party payers, and subcontractors. No matter what the transaction, there are basic questions to resolve in establishing each relationship.

Basic Questions About Any Deal

- *Who will provide the goods or services, and Who will provide payment?*
- *What exactly is each party required to do?*

- When *will each party be providing the goods or services, over what period of time, and when will payment be made?*
- Where *will the services be performed or where will the goods be delivered?*
- Why *is each party performing its obligations, and* Why *is the deal important to each party?*
- How *will satisfactory performance or delivery be measured?*
- *Does the contract address regulatory and accreditation require-ments, e.g., Medicare access to records, Medicare/Medicaid exclu-sions and sanctions, nondiscrimination, OSHA workplace safety?*
- *Does the contract address confidential information, e.g., Patient information, proprietary information and trade secrets, security and privacy of protected health information (Health Insurance Por-tability and Accountability Act [HIPAA])?*

Other Common Terms

- *Term and termination. How long with the contract last, can it be ended prior to that, and if so, how?*
- *Covenants, representations, and warranties. Will either party be asked to make promises or provide assurances to the other about, e.g., the nature of its practice or its compliance with certain laws (for example, HIPAA compliance; specifications, repair, and re-placement of goods; limitations of liability and limitations of warranty)?*
- *Services provided. These should be detailed enough so that both parties understand what is expected of them in the relationship*
- *Insurance coverage and indemnification*
- *Noncompetition*
- *Intellectual property issues. Intangible ownership rights and protec-tions are afforded to inventors, authors and businesses. Patents, trademarks, service marks, and copyrights are all types of intellec-tual property.*
  —*Ownership and licensing rights (royalties)*
  —*License to use by whom and for what purpose*
  —*Derivative works use, licensing, royalty stream*

—*Betty S. Adler*

Exemplar B.
State Government Relations and Policy and Reimbursement Issues.

Through the 1980s, academic nursing practice efforts in Pennsylvania were thwarted by many barriers to professional and advanced practice, including HMO regulations, reimbursement issues, lack of prescriptive authority, and other regulatory issues. As an educational institution graduating many types of advanced practice nurses (APNs), it was critical for the University of Pennsylvania School of Nursing (UPSON) to develop and lead an initiative to influence state regulations for APNs to practice and for patients/clients to access care by APNs. To address this need, in 1992 a small group of key UPSON faculty and supporters of care delivery by APNs began meeting to discuss strategies to address barriers to advanced nursing practice, including providing leadership to educate government agencies and leaders and helping to organize advanced practice nursing associations.

In 1995, with funding from the Independence Foundation and the Pew Charitable Trusts, a statewide educational initiative was established. The Alliance of Advanced Practice Nursing was created to educate nurses and constituents about advanced practice nursing and to address barriers to practice including in nurse managed centers and reimbursement. Key groups representing certified registered nurse practitioners (CRNPs), certified nurse midwives (CNMs), certified registered nurse anesthetists (CRNAs), and clinical nurse specialists (CNSs) began meeting and identified barriers to practice. Those barriers included lack of prescriptive authority, difficulties with reimbursement, and problems with managed-care companies credentialing CRNPs as primary care providers. As the Alliance evolved, lobbyists paid by each specialty group were included in meetings and educational sessions, and other nursing groups (nurse-managed centers, deans of schools of nursing) joined in. A grassroots network grew with an open electronic listserv contributed by UPSON and a newsletter contributed by a volunteer member. As Alliance members learned news pertinent to advanced practice nursing, this information was added to and disseminated via the listserv. Through the Alliance, a critical mass of APNs was created to lobby for supportive legislation for their practice.

In periodic updates at meetings and through e-mail, faculty members at UPSON were briefed on the Alliance's work and progress to address

APN practice barriers-at-large, as well as those UPSON was specifically experiencing in establishing its own academic practice sites. As legislation took shape at the state level (i.e., House Bill 50), the dean suggested contacting the university's Office of Commonwealth Relations ("Use" infrastructure) to ask for assistance on the state level. The director of the Office of Commonwealth Relations pledged the office's support, and the director was present for a large rally at the Capitol. One of the faculty leaders sent regular e-mail updates to the Director of the Office of Commonwealth Relations regarding hearings that were held on proposed legislation and subsequent regulations. While the director's involvement appeared at the time to have minimal impact, the visible and felt support from the university was important.

As might have been expected, opposition to the nursing legislation (PA HB 50) came from organized medicine in the state. An internal conflict at the university level was, therefore, created between the UPSON's Penn Nursing Network (PNN), practices owned and operated by the school of nursing (SON) and the University of Pennsylvania Health System (UPHS) and school of medicine. While recognizing a need to balance activities on behalf of all constituents (nursing and medicine), the Office of Commonwealth Relations did facilitate site visits by key state legislators to PNN practices. During these visits, staff and patients made the case to legislators for the need to eliminate barriers to APN practice.

—Melinda Jenkins

Exemplar C.
Federal Government Relations and Policy and Reimbursement Issues.

Academic practices are faced with a myriad of financial payment and reimbursement decisions. Yet, the creative initiatives of academic nursing practices, grounded in nursing research and innovative practice, do not easily fit into the mainstream of federal, state, and private payment structures. The ever-emerging nature of health (illness) payment structures is built on traditional physician and hospital delivery systems of care. Medicare, which represents approximately one third of the nation's *health care expenditures, dominates the language and mechanisms of payment to professionals. More important, structures in payment for advanced practice nursing that are set in the Social Security Act for Medicare are adopted by managed care and other private payers for payment of services provided by advanced practice nurses. For these reasons, it is critically important for academic nursing practices to understand federal rules of payment so that they can abide by mandated requirements and set up mechanisms of payment with managed care organizations and Medicare carriers that promote advanced practice nursing. Equally important is involving faculty in national efforts to shape reimbursement policy and participating in opportunities such as membership on national committees like the Relative-Based Relative Value System Group (RBRVS).*

When the Penn Nursing Network (PNN) was created in the early 1990s, there was no direct reimbursement for nurse practitioners via Medicare and little from Medicaid; no nurse practitioners were recognized as primary care providers (PCPs) under managed care in Pennsylvania. This had changed by the late 1990s. Currently, nurse practitioners and clinical nurse specialists are paid for their services in several ways that are dependent on their employment situation. Key points are the following:

- *Each can receive direct reimbursement from Medicare Part B (professional services)*
- *Each can negotiate with managed care organizations for terms of provider status or payment through group practices*
- *Each can be self-employed*
- *Nurse practitioners can receive direct reimbursement from Medicaid in those states using fee-for-service payment*

Because payment regulations for advanced practice nurse services have been changing incrementally for over 30 years, there is a great deal of complexity regarding rules for payment. Basic rules to keep in mind when entering into the business of providing clinical care are:

1. *Nurse practitioners and clinical nurse specialists receive direct reimbursement from Medicare for Part B services at 85% of the prevailing physician rate. A collaborative agreement with a physician is required regardless of state rules.*
2. *Nurse practitioners and clinical nurse specialists who are employed by nursing departments in Part A facilities (hospitals, home care agencies, skilled nursing facilities, hospices) cannot*

also bill Medicare Part B for services that are already covered under Part A.

3. *Nurse practitioners and clinical nurse specialists in academic medical centers are often covered by cost center charges reimbursed by Medicare and, therefore, do not bill separately.*

4. *Nurse practitioners and clinical nurse specialists have the option of billing "incident to" a physician service on a case by case basis; for these services, the practice receives 100% of the prevailing physician rate. When billing "incident to," the physician provider number is used for claims data, thus eliminating the representation of clinical nurse specialists or nurse practitioners in aggregate databases. Distinct situations limit when this billing mechanism can be used, and the provider must strictly adhere to these rules. They can only be used if the patient is "established" in the practice and not "new," and the physician must be present in the suite of practice when the service is delivered. This billing option applies to outpatient settings only and cannot be used to bill for services in emergency departments or hospitals.*

5. *Medicaid reimbursement rules vary by state, but federal rules mandate that family and pediatric nurse practitioners can bill Medicaid in a fee-for-service arrangement. As states convert Medicaid to managed care capitated systems, these rules no longer apply.*

It behooves academic practices to apprise themselves of the varying payment mechanisms that work well to cover services provided by advanced practice nurses. Because the payment system is so complex and new for APNs, a great deal of misinformation persists among billing managers, physicians, and nurses. It is essential, therefore, that information about payment in an academic practice be gathered from reliable sources that are familiar with advanced practice nursing. In addition, academic practices can challenge payers and request exemptions or special status for compensation within mandated regulations. Success of academic practices will ultimately be sustained if payment is established for their unique and quality services.

—Eileen Sullivan-Marx

REFERENCES

American Heritage Dictionary of the English Language (3rd Ed.). (1996). Boston: Houghton Mifflin Company.

Barnett, S., Niebuhr, V., & Baldwin, C. (1998). Principles for developing interdisciplinary school-based primary care centers. *Journal of School Health, 68*(3), 99–105.

Buppert, C. (1999). *Nurse practitioner's business practice and legal guide.* Gaithersburg: Aspen Publishers.

Christensen, C. (2000). *The innovator's dilemma.* New York: HarperCollins Publishers.

Eisenhardt, K., & Brown, S. (1999). Patching, restitching business portfolios in dynamic markets. *Harvard Business Review, 77*(3), 72–82.

Evans, L. K., Jenkins, M., & Buhler-Wilkerson, K. (2003). Academic nursing practice: Implications for policy. In M. D. Mezey, D. O. McGivern, & E. Sullivan-Marx (Eds.), *Nurse practitioners: Evolution of advanced practice* (4th ed., pp. 443–470). New York: Springer.

Evans, P., & Wurster, T. (2000). *Blown to bits.* Boston: Harvard Business School Press.

Foxcroft, D., Cole, N., Fulbrook, P., Jonhston, P., & Stevens, K. (2001). Organizational infrastructure to promote evidence based nursing practice (Cochrane Review). In *The Cochrane Library, Issue 3.* Oxford, UK: Update Software.

Friedman, C., Barnette, M., Buck, A., Ham, R., Harris, J., et al. (1999). Requirements for infrastructure and essential activities of infection control and epidemiology in out-of-hospital settings: A consensus panel report. *American Journal of Infection Control, 27*(5), 418–430.

Goold, M., & Campbell, A. (2002). Do you have a well-designed organization? *Harvard Business Review, 80,* 117–124.

Guarino, M. (1997). Business prospective: A complement to a successful public health agenda. *Journal of Public Health Management and Practice, 3*(4), 29–33.

Hagel, J., & Singer, M. (1999). Unbundling the corporation. *Harvard Business Review, 77*(2), 133–141.

Hamel, G. (2000). *Leading the revolution.* Boston: Harvard Business School Press.

Hardy, T. (2000). Soft landings: Dissolving a physician network. *Healthcare Financial Management, 54*(8), 66–67.

Hill, D. (2001). Physician strives to create lean, clean health care machine. *Physician Executive, 27*(5), 62.

Hoffman, P., Kline, E., George, L., Price, K., Clark, M., et al. (1995). Health care network communications infrastructure. *Proceedings of the Annual Symposium on Computer Applications in Medical Care,* 556–560.

Lang, N., & Evans, L. (1999). Forging new partnerships for financial development. In J. Ryan (Ed.), *Market-driven nursing* (pp. 115–124). Chicago: AONE/Health Forum.

Moore, G. (2000). *Living on the fault line.* New York: HarperCollins Publishers.

Neumann, C., Blouin, A., & Byrne, E. (1999). Achieving success: Assessing the role of and building a business case for technology in healthcare. *Frontiers of Health Services Management, 15*(3), 3–28.

Pardes, H. (1997). The future of medical schools and teaching hospitals in the era of managed care. *Academic Medicine, 72*(2), 97–102.

Porter, M. (1998). *Competitive strategy: Techniques for analyzing industries and competitors.* New York: Simon & Shuster.

Smith, D., & Bryant, J. (1988). Building the infrastructure for primary health care: An overview of vertical and integrated approaches. *Social Science & Medicine, 26*(9), 909–917.

Swan, B. A. (2000). Credentialing, contracting, and reimbursing nurse practitioners. *Nursing Economic$, 18*(5), 267–270.

Swan, B. A., & Cotroneo, M. (1999). Perspectives in ambulatory care: Financing strategies for a community nursing center. *Nursing Economic$, 17*(1), 44–48.

Swan, B. A., & Evans, L. (2001). Infrastructure to support academic nursing practice. *Nursing Economic$, 19*(2), 68–71.

Vincent, D., Oakley, D., Pohl, J., & Walker, D. S. (2000). Survival of nurse-managed centers: The importance of cost analysis. *Outcomes Management for Nursing Practice, 4*(3), 124–128.

West, P. (2001). Trustees and the health care infrastructure. *Trustees, 55*(1), 6.

Chapter 8

Clinical Information Systems in Support of Academic Practice, Research, and Education

Anne M. McGinley, Jeffrey Gilbert, Karen Dorman Marek, Norma M. Lang, and Lois K. Evans

Exemplar by Karen Dorman Marek

To be successful, the decision to implement a clinical information system (CIS)[1] in health care requires from the outset a vision with clear goals and objectives. A clinical information system can facilitate a variety of management, administrative, and quality management activities. Using a standardized nursing language for the systematic collection of clinical data elements related to diagnoses, nursing problems, nursing interventions, and outcome measures provides vital information about the structure, process, and outcomes of nurse-managed care (Marek, Jenkins,

---

[1]For the purposes of this chapter, clinical information system (CIS) will refer to a large computerized database management system.

Westra, & McGinley, 1998). Variations in patient problems and provider interventions can be studied, and cost-effective, innovative methods of health care delivery can be identified. Finally, information can be used in contract negotiation, education, legislative policy development, and research.

This chapter focuses on issues surrounding the development, utilization, and implementation of clinical information systems within the context of academic nursing practice. A nurse-relevant clinical-information system to support practice, clinical decision-making, and practice management provides the backdrop for a longitudinal database reflective of clinical nursing practice for use in research and evaluation of quality outcomes. The experience of the University of Pennsylvania School of Nursing's (UPSON) owned academic practices—the Penn Nursing Network (PNN)—in planning and building a CIS is presented as a primary example. Further application is provided in an exemplar from the University of Missouri. Lessons learned and strategic questions are shared to assist others in undertaking such an endeavor.

PLANNING FOR CLINICAL INFORMATION SYSTEMS

Defining Health Care Information Systems

Given the numerous overlapping terms that exist to describe health care information systems, it is important to avoid ambiguity by providing a few key definitions. Information systems use computer hardware and software to process data into information to solve problems (Hebda, Czar, & Mascara, 2001). Clinical information systems are large computerized, database management systems used to input and access data to plan, implement, and evaluate care (Axford & Carter, 1996). A nursing information system (NIS) is a type of clinical information system that supports the use and documentation of the nursing process (Hendrickson, 1993). The electronic medical record (EMR) or computer-based patient record (CPR) is an electronic repository for the longitudinal patient data typically found in the paper health care record (Andrew & Dick, 1996). In health care, administrative information systems were the first information systems to be developed. These provide demographic and financial information and are often referred to as "practice management systems" in ambulatory-care practice settings. Both clinical and administrative systems provide the capability for reporting information about patients and health care organizations.

Advantages and Disadvantages
of the Clinical Information System

A clinical information system that includes an electronic patient record has significant advantages over paper records. A clinical information system can store vast amounts of data in a small space, and the technology can support efficient data management and processing. Patient information is accessible in remote sites to many users at the same time, and information retrieval is virtually instantaneous. Newer clinical information systems can be programmed to provide a variety of clinical alerts and reminders to support clinical decision making. Use of a clinical information system can, ultimately, result in improved clinician productivity; the nature of the learning curve, however, is such that clinician time in documentation is initially increased rather than decreased. Finally, use of an electronic system can result in increased patient satisfaction because patients do not have to repeat information to multiple providers or on subsequent visits (Young, 2000).

Despite the advantages, there are some disadvantages to a clinical information system. The more obvious up-front costs associated with hardware and software acquisition and development are substantial. Other expenses related to installation, interface building, maintenance, initial and ongoing training, and evaluation may not be as readily apparent but are significant and need to be predicted.

The implementation and use of a clinical information system can result in a significant change in organizational culture. The learning curve of all participants, including the administrative leaders, needs to be considered, especially if their experience with implementation of a clinical information system is limited. Furthermore, each participant is typically at a different place in the learning curve, resulting in a need for vigilant project management.

When converting from a paper system to an electronic record, all work processes should be examined. This must occur during initial planning and reevaluated at planned intervals during and following implementation. Until a system is installed, many users have difficulty visualizing how they can work differently and be efficient with the system. The new way of working requires time and patience because implementing a CIS requires systems changes, not just substituting a computer for manual data collection methods.

If a nursing language will be used in the clinical information system, another obstacle is the lack of agreement on a standardized language to reflect nursing care. Potential users may have been educated using a variety of frameworks; thus, requesting them to use a format that is unfamiliar can cause confusion and resistance.

Finally, plans for back-up documentation need to be made in order to manage during unscheduled downtime of the system. Technical aspects associated with the implementation of a clinical information system also need to be considered, including ongoing availability of appropriate technical personnel.

Important Considerations and Challenges

Privacy, Confidentiality, and Security. Safeguarding client privacy and confidentiality has always been paramount with regard to individuals' health care information. Automation, however, has made access to client health information easier and more widespread, which has created a heightened public awareness related to the privacy and confidentiality of electronic health information. Information system security is ensured when the system and the information it stores are protected from threats of disruption. Responding to growing public concern, the federal Health Insurance Portability and Accountability Act of 1996 (HIPAA) set mandatory standards for the privacy of protected individual health information, the electronic transmissions of health information, and the security of this information (Brandt, 1995; Ettinger, 1993; Mitchell, 1993). Compliance with these standards requires significant changes to both technology infrastructure and organizational processes in all health care entities. Any plan to implement a clinical information system must incorporate the HIPAA requirements and include provisions for an ongoing quality assurance program related to the privacy, confidentiality, and security of health care information.

Documentation/Data Entry. While inputting documentation directly to the computer at the point of care provides the best, most accurate data, this may not be the most practical approach. Decisions need to be made, therefore, regarding who will enter client information (provider or support staff), when the data will be entered (during the client visit or subsequent to the visit), and in what format the data will be entered (structured form/template or free form narrative text). It is not advisable, however, for clinicians to double document, that is, first paper, then computer, since this defeats the purpose of enhancing workflow. Whenever possible, data collection should complement the users' need for information. A plan to ensure the quality and accuracy of the documentation in the clinical information system also needs to be developed as part of the ongoing quality assurance process.

All of the issues described were well thought out during planning and development of the CIS for the academic nursing practices of PNN. Advantages and disadvantages were considered and plans for documentation/ data entry were developed. Issues concerning privacy, confidentiality, and security continuously evolved during the process and required ongoing vigilance. The next section provides a description of PNN's CIS project.

CLINICAL INFORMATION SYSTEM EXPERIENCE OF PNN

Once a decision is made to go forward with plans for a clinical information system, an infrastructure plan is required that is fiscally, technically, and operationally sound (see Chapter 7). Although this chapter focuses specifically on the clinical information system, it would be remiss not to emphasize the importance of defining the more basic information technology infrastructure needs of each academic nursing practice. Other software needs are described later in this section.

The project to develop and implement a clinical information system for the practices of PNN was originally funded and supported with grants from the Philadelphia-based Independence and Scholler Foundations beginning in 1996. Ongoing support for the project was provided by the Independence Foundation through 1999. The reality is that grants do not last forever, and a plan for sustainability must be developed from the outset. Once implemented, the practices were dependent on continued operation of the clinical information system. Sustainability has been maintained by including the information technology infrastructure as part of the annual operating budget for practice (see Chapter 7).

STRATEGIC PLANNING

Choosing a System

It is essential to choose a clinical information system that will meet the needs of both the parent organization and the practice. At the time of this project's initiation, the availability of complete practice management systems was limited. Finding an acceptable system was made more complex by challenges, including the lack of a standardized nursing terminology in existing clinical information systems and system architectures that had not reached the level of sophistication and flexibility available today. Several key criteria were identified to be used in the search for PNN's clinical information system. The system had to include the elements of the Nursing Minimum Data Set (Werley & Lang, 1988) as well as a standard nursing nomenclature that captured problems, interventions, and outcomes. An intuitive design was required that was responsive to the user for the collection of data and also complemented the workflow of the nurses/clinicians. Moreover, the software had to be easily customizable so that menus could be revised and research tools could be added and deleted (Marek, Jenkins, Westra, & McGinley, 1998). The database had to be object-oriented with report-writing capability in order to generate data for operations, evaluation, and research. Last, there was a need for linkage between billing and clinical data to support ongoing operations.

After investigating several applications, a decision was made to enter into an agreement with CareFacts Information Systems, Inc. (then Epsilon Systems) to customize its existing home-care-oriented clinical software program. CareFacts Information Systems has focused on the development of community-based clinical information systems for community health and home care that are designed for the flexible capture of standardized data at the point of care by multiple disciplines in multiple settings. The CareFacts Clinical Information Management System utilizes the five steps of the nursing process—assessment, diagnosis, planning, intervention, and evaluation—as its framework for data collection and integrates the Omaha System, a classification system that uses standardized language for nursing diagnoses, interventions, and outcomes. Using relational database architecture, the CareFacts™ system includes several standardized data sets further described in the next section. Data stored in CareFacts™ are accessible by means of a custom report-writing module, which allows for the exporting of data sets in the ASCII text format. Using this feature, data can be exported to Excel and/or a statistical analysis package (e.g., SAS or SPSS) for evaluation and analysis.

At the time of the selection during the mid-1990s, CareFacts™ was a character-based, menu-driven disk operating system (DOS) program. While this structure forced users to move through the application in a specific order, the relatively simple linear flow proved to be functional for the clinicians and staff. The software has since been migrated to the Windows graphical user interface (GUI) environment, allowing for significantly greater user flexibility (see Exemplar).

Data Elements

An important component of the CIS project included the identification of key data elements to represent the problems treated, interventions performed, and outcomes sensitive to the nursing care provided. A database committee was formed to examine the needs of each practice and each discipline within each practice in order to develop flexible processes for the consistent collection of data. A number of nursing classification systems were reviewed for use in the clinical information system. The Omaha System was chosen as the standardized nursing language because of its ease of use, especially across multiple disciplines, and because it provided a useful framework for capturing the necessary data elements. The Visiting Nurses Association of Omaha developed the Omaha System. It was designed to meet the needs of community-based health providers and includes diagnoses, interventions, and outcomes (Martin & Scheet, 1992). Other classification systems needed were the International Classification of Disease's Ninth Edition Clinical Modification (ICD-9-CM), Diagnostic and Statistical Manual of Mental Disorders (DSM), and Current Procedural Terminology (CPT).

PNN is a founding member of the Regional Nursing Centers Consortium, now the National Nursing Centers Consortium, which was initiated as an association of nursing centers in Pennsylvania, New Jersey, and Delaware. An important aspect of the consortium's mission was the development of a warehouse of key data elements from member nursing centers for use in evaluation of quality and effectiveness of nurse-managed care, research, and public policy efforts (Marek, Jenkins, Westra, & McGinley, 1998; see also Chapter 12). Through small group work, common data elements were identified and defined using a format similar to that developed for the Data Elements Emergency Department Systems (DEEDS) (National Center for Injury Prevention and Control, 1997). Those data elements were also to be part of the information captured by the CareFacts™ system.

The three categories of data elements established by the Nursing Minimum Data Set (Werley & Lang, 1988) were accepted to define the data warehouse. Client descriptors included gender, race, ethnicity, date of birth, zip code, marital status, language spoken, employment status, occupation, household income, religion, and highest grade completed. Service elements were a unique identifier, date of service, time of service, payment source, type of provider, time spent in the encounter, source of referral, and site of care. Client care elements were those most useful to the practitioner and included medical diagnosis, nursing diagnosis, nursing and medical interventions, and outcomes.

DEVELOPMENT AND IMPLEMENTATION

Clinical Information System

The CARE Program. The Collaborative Assessment and Rehabilitation for Elders Program (CARE) was the first PNN practice where the CareFacts™ program was implemented. The CARE Program provided comprehensive nursing care and rehabilitation for frail elders with multiple health problems. The entire interdisciplinary team was included in the preimplementation planning process that focused on the examination and revision of the patient information to be collected using CareFacts™. Implementation of the clinical information system necessitated a close examination of the workflow of the providers. Two realities soon became clear: first, that no members of the interdisciplinary team (including nurses, physical therapists, occupational therapists, social workers, and physicians) would be able to continue to document using their original paper and pencil forms, and second, that much duplication of assessment elements existed across multiple disciplines. Through clinician involvement, The CARE Program was able to develop discipline-specific assessments resulting in acceptance of this new format for documentation. The Omaha System problems were useful in guiding identification of responsibility areas for documentation; their use also helped eliminate duplicative questions for clients and facilitated staff learning the system (Marek, Jenkins, Westra, & McGinley, 1998). Implementation of the Omaha System was very successful at The CARE Program because the change in documentation was carefully planned, training took place, and the new documentation format was initiated on paper long before a clinician touched a computer. Additionally, the Care-Facts™ system provided a mechanism to integrate research instruments as part of its data collection (e.g., Geriatric Depression Scale [GDS], Functional Independence Measure [FIM], etc.; Evans, Yurkow, & Siegler, 1995).

Multiple extensive training sessions were held for all users, led by software company personnel and PNN clinical information staff members. The clinical director and one clinical staff member were identified as "super users" and served as the primary local resources. Initially, the clinical director and her staff expressed a concern about documenting directly on the computer while sitting with a patient. Patients, however, were found to be very accepting of the activity and were actually quite interested in what was being written about them.

Health Annex. The Health Annex at the Francis J. Myers Recreation Center provides integrated primary care, women's health, and mental health services to low-income minority families (Cotroneo, Outlaw, King, & Brince, 1997). Although some of the data needs of this community-based nursing center were common to those of The CARE Program, it was necessary to make significant additional modifications to the existing Care-Facts™ program. Practitioner feedback was used to alter the program in order to facilitate the capture and retrieval of data without disrupting the usual workflow (Marek, Jenkins, Westra, & McGinley, 1998). Integrating research instruments for data collection in primary care was also possible.

Similar to The CARE Program, multiple extensive training sessions were held with clinical staff; CareFacts™ personnel and PNN clinical information staff members functioned as the trainers. In this case, the clinical director was identified as the "super user" and served as the sole local resource person.

An unexpected obstacle encountered was the difference between primary care and community nursing practice in use of the term assessment. In primary care, the Subjective-Objective-Assessment-Plan (SOAP) format was used to guide and document patient care (American Medical Association, 1997); assessment, or clinical decision-making, was based on clinical analysis of subjective and objective data by the practitioner and resulted in problem identification. In the nursing process, however, assessment encompasses only the data-gathering phase. CareFacts™ was designed according to the nursing process, so major reprogramming was needed to convert the system and its underlying architecture to support the primary-care practice format.

Additionally, the modified program format gave practitioners the choice of identifying client diagnoses from the Omaha problem list, ICD-9-CM, and/or DSM-IV. Preimplementation, the standard practice had been to use medical terms, so including Omaha problems required an additional mental and procedural step for the provider. This resulted in the application of two competing datasets, that is, medical diagnoses versus Omaha problems. This confusion was never fully resolved with a formal policy; consequently, even after implementing the electronic record, the clinicians continued to use medical diagnoses primarily without becoming proficient in the use of the Omaha System.

Other Software Needs

Consideration needs to be given to software that will be used for the required practice management functions in the event that the clinical information system chosen does not have an integrated application for this purpose. At the time of system selection, CareFacts™ did not have this billing and scheduling component, and, therefore, a separate Windows-based software package, Spectramed, was purchased to fulfill the initial practice management requirements at the Health Annex. A software program that met billing specifications for The CARE Program, which operated under Medicare as a comprehensive outpatient rehabilitation facility, was already in place. Neither Spectramed nor The CARE Program billing product had a crosswalk between the administrative and clinical applications, resulting in a need for double documentation. No further effort was made to rectify this duplicative documentation problem in The CARE Program after it closed in 1999 (see Chapter 4). For the Health Annex, it was determined (also in 1999) that the current version of the Spectramed software was not Y2K compliant. Due to changes in the ownership structure of Spectramed at that time, a decision was made to purchase an affordable off-the-shelf practice management software package product that was Y2K compliant. As a result, Medisoft Advanced Patient Accounting was installed and, as of this writing, is the billing and scheduling system in use at the Health Annex. This package handles all daily scheduling needs for multiple providers and allows for the electronic submission of billing claims. This application also has its own custom report builder augmented by Crystal Reports custom report-writing software.

Basic office productivity software is a requirement in any clinical setting and is needed to ensure that word processing, spreadsheet, and e-mail capabilities are in existence and maintained. Additionally, these products are essential for practice management and quality assurance activities. Data are only useful if there is a mechanism for evaluating the information. Applications such as Crystal Reports are useful for reporting on data in the aggregate. Statistical analysis of information obtained by reporting can be accomplished with Microsoft Excel and statistical packages such as SPSS. The open database connectivity (ODBC) standard facilitates the exchange of data between the packages described.

The vendors of most clinical information systems (e.g., CareFacts™) and practice management systems (e.g., Medisoft) require the payment of an annual maintenance or support fee. These fees can range up to 20% of the purchase cost of the applications per year and need to be included in ongoing information system budgets.

Hardware

Anyone who has ever purchased a computer for his or her use, whether personal or professional, has undoubtedly been startled by the realization that hardware requirements are constantly changing to keep pace with changing software. Regardless of the use, hardware will not last forever and needs an ongoing assessment for upgrades or replacement. Hardware typically requires a three-to-four-year replacement cycle. One might say that this is one of the largest ongoing expenses related to maintaining a clinical information system.

A network server is needed to run the clinical information system application and maintain the client data. This server, or servers (depending upon the size of the organization), should have fault-tolerant (redundant) systems to prevent the loss of mission-critical clinical data. Each of the individual PNN clinical sites, The CARE Program and the Health Annex, housed a single server for the CareFacts™ application. Network workstations should be made available at a minimum in every examining room, lab, and registration area with the consideration that these systems usually require replacement every three to four years. The Office for Research in Academic Practice (ORAP) in UPSON (see Chapter 9) was home to a third server with sufficient storage capacity to contain a data repository for the combined longitudinal clinical/research data from all practices. The CareFacts™ databases from both The CARE Program and the Health Annex were regularly replicated to this database file server.

Personnel

None of the work of this project would have been possible without adequate personnel to support the activities associated with implementing and maintaining a clinical information system. Both The CARE Program and the Health Annex at the Francis Myers Recreation Center were geographically distinct off-campus practices of PNN. As of this writing, the PNN clinical-information system project has been handled by various personnel, including a clinical information system coordinator and a database administrator. Members of the PNN clinical information project team acted as the liaisons between the clinical providers and the software developers/vendors. The clinical information system coordinator has assisted with training and support and has been responsible for the conceptual integrity of the project. The database administrator also assisted with training and was responsible for the technical integrity of the project. This person also has been responsible for hardware/software installations and the provision of ongoing on-site technical support that is available 24 hours per day, seven days per week. The team has helped facilitate research activities related to the data as well as the development and maintenance of policies and procedures for the use of CIS.

The team also had responsibilities related to ORAP (Chapter 9). These included database development and maintenance of the data repository; Web-site development and maintenance; and such organizational and administrative activities as committee work, faculty development, and grant reviews.

PNN VISION

Originators of the idea to collect nursing-relevant patient information in a longitudinal database were mavericks and sometimes paid accordingly. Many of their colleagues did not fully understand the value of having access to clinical practice data or the magnitude of the data that would be available. Once researchers realized the extent of information that was literally at their fingertips, requests for data to complete grant applications and to perform research began to appear. There were complexities, however, in incorporating those requests into an already packed work schedule for the project team, even when funds existed to offset the expenses.

While The CARE Program closed in 1999 following implementation of the Balanced Budget Act of 1997 (Evans & Yurkow, 1999), the patient information collected over a seven-year period, has provided a rich source of data for use by faculty researchers and doctoral students. The data from this practice are currently housed on a server at UPSON (see also Chapter 9).

Patient information was collected electronically at the Health Annex until 2001. At that time, upgrades and support for the DOS version of CareFacts™ were no longer available. Moreover, migration to the Windows version of CareFacts™ would have resulted in prohibitive development costs to accommodate the specific needs of primary care. Additionally, through membership in the National Nursing Centers Consortium (NNCC), an exploration was underway to implement a common Windows-based integrated EMR/practice management system across multiple nurse-managed primary care practices. Therefore, a decision was made to suspend use of CareFacts™ at the Health Annex. These data, however, remain available for use by researchers. The Medisoft practice management system continues to be used and provides demographic and utilization information for clinicians as well as researchers.

Looking to the future, work is underway to improve on the existing capture of nursing-relevant data. New technologies have been evaluated for collecting, storing, and analyzing data to improve patient care, including personal digital assistants (PDAs) and optical character recognition (OCR) scanning technology. Systems that integrate practice management functionality (i.e., billing and scheduling) with clinical information systems (or EMRs) also continue to be explored.

LESSONS LEARNED

Unified Team Vision

Implementation of a clinical information system requires a unified team vision and synchronous expectations. Differing philosophic, technologic, and financial views can interfere with evaluation of overall objectives for such a project. Setting a timeline can be fraught with complexities, but it will be helpful in meeting the deadlines associated with planning and implementation. It is essential, therefore, that the faculty and practice leaders and the technical leader function as a unit. Some of the costs include lost time and/or the use of agency personnel while the clinical staff is being trained. Project staff also often must request additional input and work from clinicians who are already very busy. Unlimited energy coupled with enthusiasm for revisions are necessities for the project team. Implementation of a clinical information system is doomed to failure without adequate resources, adequate training, and realistic expectations.

Computer and Clinical Competence

The clinical staff may have little or no advanced computer expertise, which can interfere with their understanding of the potential gains from using the clinical information system. Furthermore, software vendor representatives generally have limited current or specialized clinical experience. It is essential, therefore, that there is a team available to facilitate a clinical information system project that understands both the clinical and the technical aspects. In fact, this can help to eliminate communication difficulties due to differing professional concepts and jargon, avoid unrealistic expectations of the others' needs and capabilities, and overcome clinicians' difficulty envisioning how the proposed system will look and function.

Change in Workflow

The implementation of a clinical information system usually results in a change in workflow. This change needs to be considered during the design phase so that workflow changes can be examined prior to training. During system implementation and especially within the "go live" time frame, the clinical setting will ideally have on-site training assistance. In the absence of the ideal, at the very least, the site needs to have technical assistance readily available for on-going support. Moreover, one cannot overemphasize the need to budget adequate time for revisions, training, implementation, and re-training as needed.

Implementation Costs

Development, implementation, and maintenance of a clinical information system are costly and labor intensive. Once the clinical information system is in place, the practice will quickly come to depend on its continued operation and support. Provider involvement throughout development and implementation is essential, and ongoing training and support is vital. Consequently, the clinical information system project team, along with management, should develop a plan for sustained use of the clinical information system. It is crucial to plan for adequate financial resources, adequate personnel, and adequate time to accomplish the established goals. Provided there is adequate quality assurance, data derived from a clinical information system are far superior to that captured from paper charts.

Emerging Technologies and Regulations

Personnel should continuously scan the horizon for new technologies that can be applied to clinical information systems. PDAs, palmtops, and tablet computers are examples of the wide variety of wireless access devices currently being explored. Web-based clinical applications managed by third-party application service providers (ASPs) are now helping to reduce the technology infrastructure overhead costs for some organizations. In addition, biometric identification technologies will likely enhance the privacy and security of health information, and improved speech recognition technology will ultimately simplify the data entry process. The project team must also monitor the dynamic regulatory environment for any changes that might impact existing or proposed systems. The impact of HIPAA privacy and confidentiality regulations have yet to be fully understood, and new technological developments combined with a constantly changing political climate will likely continue to alter the regulatory landscape.

Strategic Questions to Consider

Finally, for organizations contemplating implementation and use of a clinical information system, key considerations include:

- Why implement a clinical information system? This is an important question because, given the large expense involved, a clinical information system should only be used when it is appropriate for the setting. For some settings, using a large, complex clinical information or practice management system is like using an elephant to kill an ant. If only a small amount of data is required for reporting purposes, then developing a relevant database using Access or Excel may be sufficient.
- How will the clinical data be used: for practice, for research, or both? Again, depending on the extent of data collection and/or number of data elements, a large system may be unnecessary. Also, patients need to provide informed consent for the use of their data. HIPAA requirements for obtaining this consent vary depending upon the ultimate use of the data.
- Are there specific research initiatives for which these data will be targeted? Again, this presents a need for informed consent, a defined data set, and evaluation of the most appropriate mechanism for data collection.
- Is a standard nursing classification system, for example, Omaha, Nursing Intervention Classification (NIC), Nursing Outcomes Classification (NOC), or North American Nursing Diagnosis Association (NANDA) employed in the setting? If none of these systems is currently in place, the selection and staff training and implementation of a classification system is crucial prior to its successful use in a computerized system.
- Are there any constraints to collecting patient information or sharing patient information? This is particularly important in the areas of HIV testing, family planning, and mental health.
- What is the current information system infrastructure within the organization? Without an adequate information system infrastructure, it is unlikely that implementation of a clinical system in the specific practice setting will be successful.
- What is the existing information system knowledge base within the organization? Without the ability to conduct due diligence related to investigation, implementation, and use of a clinical system, it would be impossible to plan a project of this nature.

- Can technology "champions" be identified among providers and/or support staff? As in The CARE Program and the Health Annex, additional personnel were identified to assist with training, implementation, and trouble shooting.
- What information system knowledge resources exist within the broader university setting? Although information system resources in the clinical setting or individual school may be limited, assistance from the broader university setting may provide the necessary support to initiate the investigation phase.

CONCLUSION

The PNN Clinical Information System project has proved an exciting interdisciplinary endeavor. It has brought together clinical and technical personnel as well as students, faculty, and researchers who have learned to communicate and work together to facilitate an important undertaking for PNN and UPSON. While the project has not been without challenges, lessons learned in the process have been invaluable. Next steps will involve future use of the clinical and administrative data already collected. Furthermore, training for implementation of a new, Windows-based integrated EMR/practice management system at the Health Annex is an important next step in the use of a clinical information system in the nurse-managed primary-care setting. The PNN vision has been actualized for development of a database system across practices, with common data elements— including nursing nomenclature—that serve practice, administration, and quality management as well as research and education. Vigilant strategic thinking and planning will be required in order to maintain that vision.

Exemplar.
Implementation of an integrated information system in nurse-managed community based long-term care.

University Nurses Senior Care (UNSC), a practice of the University of Missouri Sinclair School of Nursing, is a home care agency that is a licensed Medicare-certified home health agency designated as a home-and-community-based (HCB) provider for the state of Missouri. In addition, individuals ineligible for the HCB program can elect to pay out-

of-pocket to obtain services from UNSC. UNSC specializes in long-term care of the frail elderly and provides care that is different from traditional home health care, which is usually episodic and time limited. Clients of UNSC are assigned a nurse-care coordinator who monitors their health during an episode of illness and also "checks in" with them routinely to be sure that their health care needs are being met. This type of monitoring helps the nurse-care coordinator identify problems at their onset so that more severe problems can be prevented or treated early, thus, minimizing the client's health risk.

The experience of the executive director as a member of the original design and implementation team of the PNN information system project provided a major advantage in implementing CareFacts™ at UNSC. The CareFacts™ software program has its origin in home health care and was a natural fit for the practice at UNSC. UNSC uses the windows-based CareFacts™ software program that is an integrated clinical, billing, and scheduling system. In addition, the practice uses several other software products, including QuickBooks for some accounting documentation, the university-based Peoplesoft program, and Home Health Gold for financial and clinical outcome monitoring.

As a licensed home health agency, UNSC is required to collect the Outcome and Assessment Information Set (OASIS), which is used to determine payment and produces indicators for home health quality monitoring. The Omaha System framework and the OASIS data elements complement each other and are integrated into the assessment process in the CareFacts™ system. Nursing problems, interventions, and outcomes are documented using the Omaha System. In addition, since UNSC is evaluating an alternative to nursing home placement, The Minimum Data Set (MDS) is also collected so that community-based long-term care can be compared to institution-based long term care using similar case mix and quality indicators. Since many OASIS and MDS items are similar, a crosswalk was created and programmed into the data abstraction process to minimize duplicative data entry. Similar to the PNN project, data to complete the Geriatric Depression Scale (GDS), the SF-12, and the Mini Mental Status Exam (MMSE) are collected on all clients on admission and every six months.

The careful planning of the clinical data elements has enabled the creation of a longitudinal database for use in many evaluation projects. Faculties in the School of Nursing, as well as the School of Health Professions and the School of Medicine, have included UNSC as a research site for their studies. The information system at UNSC also is used in several components of student education. For example, undergraduate nursing students are exposed to use of the Omaha System and collection of mandated datasets such as OASIS and the MDS. Undergraduate and graduate students are able to aggregate data to identify common nursing problems in different populations so that they can target interventions in various quality improvement projects. Finally, the longitudinal database provides fertile ground for doctoral students to experience large database research with a variety of clinical and administrative datasets.

The next step in computerization of UNSC is home health-aide documentation. UNSC is currently planning use of personal digital assistants (PDAs) by the home health aides to streamline the massive paperwork shuffle that accompanies each home health aide visit. The software for the PDAs will be integrated into the CareFacts™ system. Other projects in the planning stage are the MD.2 medication administration machine for clients requiring medication management services. This system administers medications on a specified time schedule and will notify UNSC by the client's phone line if a dose is missed.

UNSC is successful in part due to the integrated information system it has tailored for its use over the past four years. Each new software implementation has required changes in the staff's workflow processes; the staff at UNSC believes, however, that each new product has produced more positives than negatives once it is fully implemented.

—*Karen Dorman Marek*

REFERENCES

American Medical Association (1997). *CPT 97.* Chicago: Author.

Andrew, W., & Dick, R. (1996). On the road to the CPR: Where are we now? *Healthcare Informatics, 17*(5), 48–52.

Axford, R., & Carter, B. (1996). Impact of clinical information systems on nursing practice. *Computers in Nursing, 14*(3), 156.

Brandt, M. (1995). CPR alert: Ten steps to end the great paper chase. *Healthcare Informatics, 12*(2), 105–108.

Cotroneo, M., Outlaw, F., King, J., & Brince, J. (1997). Integrated primary health care. *Journal of Psychosocial Nursing, 35*(10), 21–27.

Ettinger, J. E. (1993). Introduction: Key issues in information security. In J. E. Ettinger (Ed.), *Information security: Applied information technology* (pp. 1–10). London: Chapman & Hall.

Evans, L. K., & Yurkow, J. (1999). Balanced budget of 1997: Impact on a nurse managed academic nursing practice for frail elders. *Nursing Economics, 17*(5), 280–282, 297.

Evans, L. K., Yurkow, J., & Siegler, E. (1995). The CARE Program: A nurse-managed collaborative outpatient program to improve function of frail older people. *Journal of the American Geriatric Society, 43,* 1155–1160.

Hebda, T., Czar, P., & Mascara, C. (2001). *Handbook of informatics for nurses and health care professionals, 2nd ed.* Upper Saddle River, NJ: Prentice-Hall.

Hendrickson, M. (1993). The nurse engineer: A way to better nursing information systems. *Computers in Nursing, 11*(2), 67–71.

Marek, K. M., Jenkins, M., Westra, B. L., & McGinley, A. M. (1998). Implementation of a clinical information system in nurse-managed care. *Canadian Journal of Nursing Research, 30*(1), 37–44.

Martin, K. S., & Scheet, N. J. (1992). *The Omaha System: Applications for community health nursing.* Philadelphia: W. B. Saunders.

Mitchell, C. J. (1993). Management of secure systems and security within OSI. In J. E. Ettinger (Ed.), *Information security: Applied information technology* (pp. 47–60). London: Chapman & Hall.

National Center for Injury Prevention and Control (1997). *Data elements for emergency department systems.* Release 1.0. Atlanta: Centers for Disease Control and Prevention.

Werley, H., & Lang, N. M. (1988). *Identification of the Nursing Minimum Data Set.* New York: Springer.

Young, K. M. (2000). *Informatics for healthcare professionals.* Philadelphia: F. A. Davis.

Chapter 9

Integrating Research and Practice

Lois K. Evans, Norma M. Lang, and Barbara Medoff-Cooper

Exemplar by Linda H. Aiken

Access to clinical settings that utilize the best evidence-based practices is essential for educating the next generation of nurses. Identifying and solving problems rooted in clinical practice necessitates the thoughtful, critical eye of the clinician-scholar and the collaboration of the researcher. To advance the science of nursing, a creative interweaving of the three arms of the tripartite mission is required, such that knowledge to solve practice problems is evolved from research, disseminated in the classroom, and tested in the clinical arena in an interrelated fashion—each component reliant on and informing the other. Academic nursing practices that embrace "the intentional integration of education, research and clinical care" (Lang, Evans, & Swan, 2002, p. 63) can provide just the environment for achieving these goals.

One aim of the University of Pennsylvania School of Nursing (UPSON) has been that each component of its academic nursing practices will be research based and research generating. The purpose for academic nursing practice initiatives is not only to enrich the school's educational offerings and ensure the provision of quality clinical care, but also to produce knowledge for advancing the discipline. At UPSON, a major strategy for achieving these goals had been the appointment of faculty to clinical, administrative, and research facilitation positions in partner/affiliate practices (e.g., University of Pennsylvania Health System, Children's Hospital of Philadelphia, and Visiting Nurse Association of Greater Philadelphia), a model in place since the 1980s. As UPSON took increasing responsibility for developing its own network of prototypic community-based practices in the 1990s, however, the need for more visible and substantive resources and strategies to further support such integration was identified. This chapter describes one such resource, the Office for Research in Academic Practice (ORAP), as it was first conceived, partially implemented and re-envisioned over a five-year period. The effectiveness of strategies implemented through the ORAP to stimulate research in UPSON's academic nursing practices is evaluated, and future directions are discussed. An exemplar further explicates the richness of academic nursing practice-research linkage.

OFFICE FOR RESEARCH IN ACADEMIC PRACTICE (ORAP): A STRATEGIC RESOURCE

Background

Most schools of nursing that embark on academic nursing practice development identify their intent to facilitate faculty research as well as to provide educational sites for students and quality health care to a specified population. The inclusion by educational programs of innovative practices for use as learning laboratories has its own set of challenges. These include low patient volumes, physical space restrictions, and limited numbers of preceptors which may preclude satisfactory student placements. The integration of research within these innovative practices, however, is perhaps even more challenging (Jones & Van Ort, 2001; Macnee, 1999; Sawyer, Alexander, Gordon, Juszczak, & Gillis, 2000; Taylor & Marion, 2000, Evans, Swan, & Lang, 2003). In many academic nursing practice settings, especially those that are innovative models, the conduct of clinical research using traditional methods is hampered by limited patient enrollments or caseloads, which results in small potential sample size for any particular age or population group. The lack of comparable sites for evaluating overall program outcomes is also often a restrictive factor. Further, unless the practice is serving a population or demonstrating an intervention that holds research interest for specific faculty members, capturing the "scholarly attention" of non-clinical faculty for collaborative research is difficult (Grey & Walker, 1998; Grey,1999). Finally, few affiliated, faculty- or school-of-nursing-operated community-based practices have an existing database that includes nursing language and/or common data elements that would facilitate cross-practice research. Utilizing clinical practice data for health services and outcomes research is necessarily constrained by each of these characteristics.

As described previously (see Chapters 2 & 5), the evolution of academic nursing practice at UPSON has occurred in three overlapping phases. First, in the 1980s, was the formalization of academic nursing practice by creating a new standing faculty role, that of the clinician educator (CE). Through CE appointments in health care organizations, the dean and faculty facilitated a second phase, the development of strong affiliations and partnerships. This phase focused on building evidence-based professional practice environments (Fagin, 1986; see Chapter 5). More recently, UPSON opened its own network of community-based practice sites under an umbrella called the Penn Nursing Network (PNN). As UPSON embarked on this third phase of academic nursing practice development, a vision for research integration for all of its practices was shaped. The school planned the systematic description, study, and evaluation of academic nursing practices, specifically their impact on clients, families, communities, and providers. The intent (see Exemplar) was to derive evidence-based care guidelines, demonstrate best practice models, and inform public policy regarding the quality of advanced practice nursing care (Colling, 1993; Lang, 1995; Lang, Jenkins, Evans, & Matthews, 1996; Joint Task Force, 1993; UPSON 1993, 1995; see also Chapter 4).

As the number of individual faculty with programs of funded research has grown, so has UPSON's success in supporting continued faculty research development through establishment of research centers; first, a generic center for nursing research and then centers focused on specific programs or subject areas (e.g., initially nursing history, health policy, serious illness, low–birth weight infants; see www.nursing.upenn.edu/research for current centers). Eager to circumvent some of the aforementioned impediments to the integration of research and practice, UPSON sought to identify a visible space in which to concentrate its academic nursing practice-related research efforts. A grant from the university's Research Facilities Development Fund enabled renovation of space for this purpose in the Nursing Education Building, which houses UPSON. The proposal envisioned a system for linking the campus with off-site community-based practices that would produce a central pool of administrative and clinical data for use in research and evaluation. The plan was to develop a common database for these linked practices and a data repository that could be shared by faculty to permit comparisons across settings, testing of interventions, evaluation research, and the educational preparation of students in information science and technology in support of evidence-based health care (see Fig. 9.1). The resultant suite housed three private offices, open receptionist and data-entry work areas, a medium-sized conference room, and a computer room with 10 work stations. It was anticipated that research assistants and students working on individual research or educational projects would use the workstations, utilizing the repository data, including datasets from clinical records and other clinical research projects.

The ORAP space was officially dedicated with a ribbon-cutting ceremony in fall, 1997. ORAP was heralded as a resource for UPSON investigators, clinicians, and students to facilitate and catalyze increased research effort based in PNN and other faculty practices. Its three functions were to serve as

- A repository for clinical, administrative and financial data related to academic nursing practice
- A focal point for continuing work on nursing clinical database development using common nursing language and data elements
- The operations center for quality management and evaluation functions for the PNN practices

ORAP was envisioned primarily as an important link between research and practice rather than as a stand-alone center per se. It, therefore, provided a complementary support function that required a sense of *shared ownership* by both practice and research, a key feature that was facilitated through ORAP's coleadership by the directors of the Center for Nursing Research and Academic Nursing Practice.

EARLY DEVELOPMENT

Governance

The directors of the Center for Nursing Research and of Academic Nursing Practice shared interests in practice-based research. Responsibility for activ-

Education

✓Curricula for information-based Health Care

✓Student Applications for Data Use (Clinical)

✓Student Applications for Data Use (Research)

Research

✓Health Services Research

✓Health Policy Research

✓Population-Based Studies

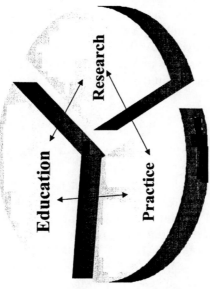

Practice Support

✓Information Systems Services

✓Quality Management Services

✓Negotiation of Reimbursement
  with Payers

FIGURE 9.1   Contribution of ORAP to tripartite mission.

ities related specifically to the quality management and evaluation of the school-owned PNN practices were delegated to the director of Academic Nursing Practices. The director of the Center for Nursing Research was responsible for activities specifically related to oversight and facilitation of academic nursing practice research. While a formal faculty advisory council was provided for in the planning, it was never formed. Instead, an UPSON Academic Practice Research Review Committee was convened soon after the creation of ORAP. The committee's purpose was to review and monitor research proposals from faculty, staff, or doctoral students wishing to conduct research involving PNN and its resources (i.e., clinical staff, clients/families, and clinical and/or administrative records). Essentially this process provided for the systematic review of research proposals for feasibility and subject or site burden, but not for scholarly merit. The UPSON practice committee reviewed and distributed procedural and related documents.

Fiscal Support, Staffing, and Strategic Planning

To finance practice infrastructure adequately, including evaluation/research and clinical information systems development, support at the multi-million-dollar level was initially sought from several philanthropic sources. Although well-conceived, these large-scale efforts had only limited success, and neither the overall infrastructure nor ORAP was ever fully operationalized as originally conceived. On the other hand, obtaining support for specific project-related infrastructure proved more opportune in financing ORAP. For example, some infrastructure and support for evaluation of outcomes were built-in components of the William Penn Foundation grant that underwrote the establishment of the Collaborative Assessment & Rehabilitation for Elders (CARE) Program and the HRSA Division of Nursing Special Projects grant for initiation of the Health Annex, a community-based nursing and primary care center. The first successfully funded major project specifically for infrastructure was for development of a clinical information system and database for the Penn Nursing Network practices, supported by the Philadelphia-based Independence Foundation (see also Chapters 8 & 12). Thus, ORAP initially housed the faculty and staff responsible for developing and maintaining this clinical information system and data repository. Foundation funding from the Josiah Macy Jr. Foundation in support of academic nursing practice dissemination also helped underwrite appropriate aspects of ORAP's work. Between-grant support was provided by the operating budget of the Penn Nursing Network, fees charged to researchers requesting development of clinical datasets from the repository, and consultation provided by staff to other schools of nursing. In its fourth year of operation, a strategic planning process for ORAP was initiated to reconfigure its mission and niche, as well as to identify potential sources of ongoing funding.

Work Focus

From the outset, the types of research questions envisioned for exploration through the resources of ORAP included the following:

- *Description or nursing's academic nursing practices:* Who is being served, and what are their needs?
- *Process of care delivery:* What do nurses and staff do with and for clients, and how do they do it?
- *Cost & Quality Outcomes:* What difference does it make, and at what cost?

For PNN practices, faculty directors for each practice developed with their teams a written research agenda in concert with the practice model and population(s) served. In turn, this guided the selection of clinical assessment and monitoring instruments as well as tools for use in the practice, and it helped focus faculty on potential funding opportunities. In addition, UPSON's practice committee appointed a two-year group called the Working Group on Education, Practice, and Research Integration. This group identified areas for concentration, including identification of common data elements and strategies to encourage and facilitate intra- and interdisciplinary and interpractice connections for research. It was hoped that the resulting common data collection tools and, eventually, the common data elements, would be shared across the school's academic nursing practices—not only those of PNN, but those of individual CE faculty as well.

IMPLEMENTATION AND OUTCOMES

ORAP was conceived to support integration of the tripartite mission in academic nursing practice (Fig. 9.1). From ongoing dialogue on how best to achieve this goal, several of the following strategies evolved over the five-year period reported here.

Practice Support

PNN clinical information system and database development. As mentioned earlier, at the same time that space was being renovated for ORAP, UPSON was developing an integrated and networked computerized clinical and practice management information system with funding from the Independence Foundation (Marek, Jenkins, Westra, & McGinley, 1998). This system was intended to communicate point-of-service information from each of the participating clinical practices to a central repository housed in ORAP. A detailed description of the information system and its development can be found in Chapter 8. ORAP staff provided PNN reports and access to clinical and administrative data that PNN faculty directors and staff required for preparing stewardship reports for existing grants and for developing new grant proposals. For example, ORAP staff provided data necessary to identify common clinical problems among patient populations, verify sufficient potential sample size, and so on. In addition, the support from the Independence Foundation permitted UPSON to bring together nurses and faculty from several community-based nursing centers in the Philadelphia region to begin to develop a set of common data elements and definitions that would facilitate collaborative research among these centers. Thus, it was hoped that two of the problems enumerated earlier in this chapter, namely, the small size of innovative practices and the lack of a clinical information system with common nursing language and data elements, could be prevented or solved. As described in Chapter 8, the road to implementation of a data system in two of the PNN practices, the community-based nursing center (Health Annex) and The CARE Program, was bumpy, yet one rich in new learning. Knowledge was gained about the selection and modification of an electronic clinical information system for community-based nursing practices, the challenges of selecting a system that can be used in a wide range of practice sites, the problems associated with Internet conveyance of data and privacy and confidentiality issues. The last has served PNN well in preparing for upcoming implementation of the privacy aspects of the Health Insurance Portability and Accountability Act (HIPAA).

Other data sets and resources housed in ORAP. In addition to controlled clinical and practice administrative data, ORAP provided student and faculty access to the Philadelphia Health Management Corporation's regional household health survey data, available through PNN's membership in the National Nursing Centers Consortium. Students, especially those in community health nursing courses, and faculty interested in doing needs assessments to support new program proposals utilize this dataset regularly. Other resources that have been made available in ORAP include the Agency for Healthcare Research and Quality's (AHRQ) Computerized Needs-Oriented Quality Measurement Evaluation System (CONQUEST) program; resource files and reference texts regarding quality management, community nursing centers, academic nursing practice, and nursing classification systems; and student-developed electronic tables of evidence regarding common clinical problems. Finally, ORAP maintained the UPSON Academic Nursing Practice website, including design and updating of features and content for the overall PNN and individual practice sites, other faculty practices, linkages to practice partners and affiliates, and the Penn Macy Initiative to Advance Academic Nursing Practice.

Education Outcomes

ORAP provided support to a number of student-driven research projects in PNN practices, both team and independent. At least one undergraduate presented a peer-reviewed poster on her project at a national meeting (Glancey & Sochalski, 1999). Since 2000, senior nursing students have deposited in ORAP their senior inquiry papers, including tables of evidence, for use by clinicians and others in a beginning attempt to contribute to building the evidence base for common practice problems. Nurse-practitioner students participated in a pilot project to classify nursing diagnoses and interventions in their practice using a range of recording mechanisms developed in collaboration with ORAP staff (Jenkins, 2002). And doctoral and undergraduate students alike have amassed unique informatics experience through part-time employment in ORAP.

The information-related aspects of ORAP's goals were slower to evolve, in part because of the effort expended to develop integrated clinical information systems. Nonetheless, the clinical information system development work provided UPSON a place at the table when an interdisciplinary Center for Health Informatics at the University of Pennsylvania was commencing. Faculty involvement in this interschool center was instrumental in supporting postdoctoral study for nurses in informatics and in launching a track in nursing clinical informatics at the masters and doctoral levels. These informatics students have already used, with approvals, clinical datasets housed in ORAP to facilitate their learning.

Research Facilitation

ORAP staff facilitated several faculty research projects, preparing datasets from electronic patient data. For example, the longitudinal research project funded by National Institute for Nursing Research and National Institute on Aging to evaluate the outcomes of one of PNN's early practices, The CARE Program (Sochalski, 2001), required ORAP staff assistance in electronic data retrieval. Other studies (for example, depressive symptoms among frail elders of African descent) have also been conducted using datasets constructed from The CARE Program electronic clinical records, following approval by the University of Pennsylvania Institutional Review Board. Although now closed (Evans & Yurkow, 1999), the six years of CARE Program clinical and administrative data were retained in ORAP. Two doctoral students are currently accessing these data for their research, one studying dependency among frail elders and one examining characteristics and outcomes of cognitively impaired elders undergoing rehabilitation. ORAP staff also supported conduct of a study of depressive symptoms and their correlates in a population of chronically ill adult women of African descent that is served by the community-based nursing center (Health Annex).

The volume of requests from faculty or doctoral students to access the PNN practices for research remains small; for example, in the calendar year 2001–2002, only three such requests were processed by the Academic Practice Research Review Committee. This reflects, in part, that growth in volume and systems maturation of PNN practices was necessary to fully support research. On the other hand, faculty were slow to appreciate the potentially rich resources of these practices for research. Also lacking was a strong interest from a broad range of faculty in the use of nursing language as different from and complementary to the usual classification systems found in health care (International Classification of Diseases [ICD], Current Procedural Practice Terminology [CPT], Diagnostic and Statistical Manual of Mental Disorders [DSM]) and with which they were more familiar.

Several strategies to bridge the research–practice chasm were used over the five-year period; all were attempts to increase readiness of faculty and clinicians for joint research endeavors. Four of these are briefly described.

"Conversations with Norma Lang." As the clinical information system that incorporated a nursing language and data elements was being initiated in the PNN practices (see Chapter 8), it became clear that faculty and clinical staff would need to understand and embrace it to take full advantage of the research and practice opportunities that such a system afforded (Coenen, Marek, & Lundeen, 1996; Marek, 1997; Baernholdt & Lang, 2003). With ready availability of an internationally renowned leader in nursing language and classification (Lang, 1995), ORAP convened a series of "Conversations with Norma Lang" that focused on the importance of nursing language in naming and describing the work of nurses in order to measure its cost and quality outcomes. Three sessions—"Why nursing data?", "What nursing data?", and "Where nursing data?"—were held. The session locations were rotated between UPSON's Nursing Education Building and PNN clinical settings, and the times were varied (early morning, lunchtime, end of day) in order to accommodate both faculty and clinical staff schedules. Attendance by faculty, clinicians and students at these "conversations" was excellent and the dialogue robust. Interest was piqued, especially among master clinicians and clinician-educator faculty. Presence was not as high, however, for faculty engaged primarily in research. While some faculty and doctoral candidates (Naylor, Bowles, & Brooten, 2000; Bowles, 2000) had undertaken research using nursing classification, a general lack of awareness among faculty existed of its potential for their work (see also Chapter 8).

Research Think Tanks. Sessions cosponsored by the Practice Committee Work Group on Research, Education and Practice Integration, ORAP, and the relevant research center(s) in the school built awareness among faculty and clinicians about opportunities associated with PNN practices and practices of individual faculty members. The aim was to generate opportunities for research-practice linkages in areas of mutual interest. Each clinician-educator and the leadership team (practice director-faculty academic director) for each relevant PNN practice presented an overview of their practice, and the research center director presented a brief overview of the center's research interests. Because of the concentration and greater maturity of gerontologic-focused practices in PNN and elsewhere (see Exemplar B, Chapter 5), the first think tank logically focused on opportunities in aging. Faculty in the Center for Gerontologic Nursing Science, clinician-educator faculty engaged in practice with elders, and leaders and staff from the four PNN practices that were providing services to older adults at that time were invited to attend. The second think tank focused on maternal and child research in academic nursing practices; it involved faculty from two research centers (the Center for Research for Women, Children & Families and the Center for Urban Health Studies), ORAP, clinician-educators in maternal child practices, and faculty and clinicians from the three PNN practices providing services to these populations. The think tank on care of elders, while enthusiastically received, was convened and attended by gerontologic nursing faculty already knowledgeable about the PNN practice opportunities because they had also helped to design, direct, advise, and practice in them. The opposite was true, however, for the maternal/child think tank. No research center faculty were then engaged or interested in research that matched the settings or populations available in PNN, and none had been involved in establishing these practices. Thus, stimulating a "match" was challenging. The time required for percolating ideas and the need for repetitive opportunities for dialogue cannot be understated, however. Although no immediate outcomes were observable, over time at least two research projects evolved (depression in the aged and in childbearing women) that had likely been spurred by these think tanks.

Funding for Pilot Projects. Faculty who held established positions in partner and affiliated practice sites (Hospital of the University of Pennsylvania, Children's Hospital of Philadelphia, Visiting Nurse Association of Philadelphia) already had a history of conducting research in those settings (see, for example, Barnsteiner, Ford, & Howe, 1995; Brown, Meier, Spatz, Zukowshy, & Spitzer, 1996; Dansky, Palmer, Shea, & Bowles, 2001; Grey, Lipman, & Cameron, 1997; Houldin, Jacobsen, & Lowery, 1996; Kagan et al., 2002; Kurlowicz, 2001; O'Sullivan & Jacobsen, 1992; Richmond, Kauder, & Schwab, 1998; Stringer, 1998). The research of several tenure-track faculty had also been facilitated by UPSON's strong academic partnership or affiliations with select clinical agencies (for example, Brooten et al., 1986; Gennaro, Fehder, Nuamah, Campbell, & Douglas, 1997; Gennaro, Fehder, & York, 1997; McCorkle et al., 2000; Medoff-Cooper, McGrath, & Bilker, 2000; Naylor et al., 1994; Strumpf & Evans, 1988). None of the established affiliated sites, however, had yet incorporated a nursing classification system in its database as had some of those in the PNN. Recognizing the relative ease of conducting research in large agencies with supportive infrastructure and high patient volume, compared with smaller and less established practice sites like those of the PNN, an attempt was made to prime the pump, so to speak. To generate research in the PNN practices, a small fund was made available from the PNN budget to support pilot studies on evidence-based care. The request for proposals (RFP) emphasized that preference would be given to studies involving PNN practices (especially its information system) that had likelihood for future larger scale funding. A mechanism for independent pilot proposal review already in place in the UPSON was used. Unfortunately, none of the few applications submitted proposed to use PNN data or practice sites.

Nursing Grand Rounds and Academic Nursing Practice Rounds. A public forum was conceived in which larger groups of faculty and clinicians would have access to the thinking about the values of deliberately integrating research and practice. In ORAP's third year, it cosponsored with the Nursing Service of the University of Pennsylvania Health System (UPHS) a series of Nursing Grand Rounds that focused on practice problems of interest to faculty and clinical staff alike. In years 4 and 5, ORAP held a focused series of four Academic Nursing Practice Rounds, cosponsored with nursing service at UPHS, UPSON's Practice Committee, and relevant research centers. Topics were chosen to reflect both community-based and institution-based practice problems that would be of broad interest to and attract clinicians, clinician-educators, and researchers to the dialogue. Aimed at highlighting the deliberate integration of research and practice, the topics included depression in primary care, evidence-based practice with specialty populations, faculty-clinician collaboration to improve pediatric care, impact of the prospective payment system on home care utilization and quality, complementary therapies, evidence-based staff retention strategies, documentation of outcomes in computerized primary care records, and injury prevention and outcomes. These academic nursing practice rounds were increasingly well attended and positively evaluated, and speaker slides were placed on the academic nursing practice website for access by a broader audience. At least one doctoral study, on effects of prospective payment policy on psychiatric home care for older adults, evolved from the dialogue.

RE-EVALUATION AND RECONFIGURATION OF ORAP AS A RESOURCE

As the practices of individual UPSON faculty and PNN have changed over time, so the thinking has evolved about efficacious ways to facilitate research integration. Barriers to goal achievement included lack of sufficient or targeted funding for ORAP, competing agendas for the ORAP faculty leaders, changes in the practice configuration and infrastructure, and lack of readily identifiable comparison sites for evaluating these model practices.

As mentioned earlier, specific funded projects, such as clinical information system development, quality management, practice-related web projects, and participation in academic nursing practice dissemination, were related to the overall aims of ORAP and indirectly supported its work. Each of these efforts was important in helping to provide the underpinnings for research and practice integration. None, however, had integration per se as its major goal. And since programs follow funding, the resultant diffusion of effort and focus made it difficult for ORAP to fully achieve its aims.

The idea of codirection of ORAP from leaders of the two related areas, research and practice, made logical sense, yet that, too, fell short of expectations. Role-specific agendas that competed for time from each of these leaders made it difficult to commit concentrated effort on ORAP development. And, given the importance of clinical database development and management to achieving ORAP goals, the leaders' own acknowledged lack of expertise and interest in health care informatics was an obstacle. Those UPSON faculty who had informatics expertise were fully engaged in other work or were junior faculty, and timely recruitment of senior faculty who could seek funding for practice-based research and lead this initiative proved challenging.

Finally, awareness was slow to develop that no single commercial product was likely to meet the needs of each of the distinct and diverse types of practices in PNN. These ranged from a community-based practice that provided integrated primary, mental health, and women's health services within a public health model (Health Annex/Health Corner; see chapter 11), to a specialty women's health practice for institutionalized women (Hamburg), to nurse-midwifery practices. Others included an integrated acute and long-term care model for the frail elderly (Living Independently For Elders (see Exemplar B, Chapter 5) and a provider/institution-focused consultation service (Gerontologic Nursing Consultation Service, see Exemplar B, Chapter 5). This, together with the contraction of PNN practices that occurred in the late 1990s (see Chapter 4 & Table 5.2 in Chapter 5), further challenged the resources for developing an integrated data system across all PNN practices. Additionally, the time required to achieve faculty consensus on common data elements and data sharing was underestimated. Yet, the identification of and commitment to a set of defined common data elements and categories to be collected in all practices, regardless of type, remains prudent for the ongoing conduct of research within the full range of UPSON's academic nursing practices. For this goal to be achieved, efforts will need to be revitalized and will have to include faculty commitment to share access to research and clinical datasets.

Several new solutions are being developed to address the challenges associated with conducting evaluation research in small unique practices without easily identifiable comparison sites. For example, The CARE Program, a unique and innovative interdisciplinary rehabilitation program for the frail elderly, had no identifiable comparable sites to use for the outcomes evaluation. Thus, an evaluation plan that utilized large national datasets to create a randomized comparison group was developed that holds promise as a new methodology for similar evaluations (Sochalski, 2001).

Likewise, the linkage of the PNN's relatively small community-based nursing center (Health Annex) to other nursing centers of similar size through its membership in the National Nursing Centers Consortium will facilitate the eventual conduct of larger scale research. The ongoing work, begun at Penn and continued in the NNCC Data Project (Marek, Jenkins, Westra, & McGinley, 1998), to collect a set of common data elements among member centers using an electronic point-of-service health care record will also be useful on a national basis as other nursing centers affiliate to conduct research and outcome studies (see also Chapter 12). Sensibly, faculty academic directors for Living Independently For Elders (LIFE), UPSON's Program of All-inclusive Care for the Elderly (PACE), plan to link with other PACE programs through the national PACE providers organization to mount evaluation studies.

At the same time, faculty are conducting research on health-related quality of life to compare the experiences of LIFE members with that of elders enrolled in other long-term care models regionally (Naylor & Buhler-Wilkerson, 1999). And faculty practicing with small caseloads of children, or adolescents, or breastfeeding moms, or the seriously mentally ill would do well to link with similar practices through mechanisms such as the practice-based research network (Deshefy-Longhi, Swartz, & Grey, 2002) to conduct research more easily. The notion of an academic nursing practice research alliance (see Chapter 12) holds promise for providing similar access on a national basis for faculty in research-intensive universities. Again, commitment to nursing language and a set of common data elements is critical to reaching the full potential of describing the outcomes of these practices.

A structure like ORAP can serve many important roles: creating and housing clinical and other large datasets for research access, facilitating think tanks to generate research questions and methodologies, providing the focal point for informatics education for nursing and other health sciences students, and housing evidence-based practice resources. At UPSON, several specific new strategies have been recommended for future exploration that would further exploit the gains made by the ORAP structure:

- *Meta Data Dictionary*. Development of a meta data dictionary that includes the description of data elements and their properties from existing research and clinical datasets in UPSON would facilitate the use of secondary data to answer new research questions.
- *Dataset and Resource Repository*. Providing a house for clinical, large reference (e.g., Medicare, Magnet Hospital, community survey), and selected research data sets as well as search tools and resources would facilitate access and utilization by a larger number of investigators.
- *Tables of Evidence*. Making available categorized student-developed tables of evidence in support of evidence-based practice would provide access by clinicians in practice who are working on guideline development. It also would encourage subsequent cohorts of graduate and undergraduate students to continue to develop common themes.
- *Evidence-base Development*. Work begun by two postdoctoral students on evidence-base building, with direct linkage to the Campbell Collaborative, is another way that a resource like ORAP could support development of capacity in evidence-based care in nursing.
- *Dissemination*. Evidence dissemination that began in UPSON's summer Penn Macy Institute for Advancing Academic Nursing Practice *Building the Evidence Base* can be continued through efforts of relevant research centers and PNN's *PNNConsulting/GNCS*.

While the original strategies envisioned for ORAP to complement and support UPSON's academic nursing practice agenda have, of necessity, changed, ample opportunity remains for it, or its progeny, to continue to meet goals of research-practice integration that are essential to academic nursing practice success.

SUMMARY AND CONCLUSIONS

Several potential solutions to the research integration challenge have been identified in the literature these include development of practice-based research networks; congruence in faculty practice, teaching and research foci; collaboration between and among research and clinical faculty; consistency with a given practice over time; and congruence between practice models and research agendas supported by development of a minimum dataset (Deshefy-Longhi, Swartz, & Grey, 2002; Brown, 2001; Fagin, 2000; Jones & VanOrt, 2001; Mayhew, 1994; Macnee, 1999, Naylor & Buhler-Wilkerson, 1999; Zachariah & Lundeen, 1997). In testament to a dedicated and excellent staff, successes of the Office for Research in Academic Practice at the University of Pennsylvania School of Nursing have been forged despite a limited budget, lack of consistent faculty leadership, and a continual set of hurdles to be overcome. Each trial, whether successful for not, has clearly contributed to building awareness and enhancing a valuing for academic nursing practice within the school, a necessary prerequisite to the integration of research with practice. In retrospect, here are a few lessons learned about research integration facilitation strategies that appear to work, at least in an environment like UPSON:

- *Link practices to specific research centers or teams.* Examples at UPSON are LIFE linked with the Center for Gerontologic Nursing Science, the Hartford Center of Geriatric Nursing Excellence, and the Health Annex linked with the Center for Health Outcomes and Policy Research. Research projects are ongoing in each of these practices by faculty engaged in the relevant research center.
- *Academic Nursing Practice Rounds.* These seminars hold promise as another way to bring awareness to faculty and clinical staff of common research problem areas and evolving evidence bases. They may also serve over time to link potential researchers and practicing clinicians for new projects.
- *Publication of descriptive work.* Recalling that careful description lays the groundwork for research, faculty should be encouraged to publish articles that describe their practices. In a 10-year period, for example, UPSON faculty and clinician colleagues published nearly 60 articles describing the academic nursing practices of the PNN alone (Evans, 2001).
- *A cheerleader or matchmaker.* No single person can accomplish research integration, yet such a champion is essential for providing linkages and "bringing the horses to water."

Continuing assessment of the role of research-practice-education integration in the daily fabric of a research-intensive environment is required to "get it right" in any given setting. Given the importance of context and environment, each school of nursing will necessarily organize differently to achieve the goals of integrating research with academic nursing practice. The University of Pennsylvania School of Nursing's Office of Research and Practice is one example of how a visible "connector" for practice and research is an important ingredient in achieving the academic nursing practice mission.

ACKNOWLEDGMENTS

The authors wish to acknowledge the intellectual and literary contributions of Kathleen Welsh Beveridge, whose dogged pursuit of financial support for these efforts contributed greatly to the evolution of the Office for Research in Academic Practice.

Exemplar.
Academic Practice: A Rich Laboratory for Nursing Research.

As Dorothy Smith (1971), nursing leader and former dean at the University of Florida, once stated, "To produce [a] second Florence Nightingale, there will need to be a different kind of education . . . the scientific study of the nursing problems of patients. . . . " Pursuing nursing's research agenda to improve health care for individuals, families, and communities requires that nursing act deliberately to impact systems of care, caring interventions, and health care policy. Where better to spearhead these initiatives than in schools of nursing in research-intensive universities with their rich mix of seasoned research and practice faculty? In these environments, some of the highest priorities for nursing today can be solved: organizational reforms in hospitals, access to primary care, viability of academic health centers, caring for the underserved, and reinventing public health nursing.

Schools of nursing that have integrated missions can more easily mount the types of collaborations among many people required to undertake such research, disseminate the findings, and form a research culture or presence in which each feeds the other. A school such as the University of Pennsylvania School of Nursing has certain advantages for such research development. These include owning its own academic nursing practices and databases, having access to data from other systems with which it is associated, and cultivating strong affiliations with a university health system and other hospitals and health care agencies that have large databases. Among other assets are the existence of university research facilities, scholarly practices of clinician-educator faculty in a variety of settings, strong departments and faculty in behavioral and social sciences, top-ranked professional schools contiguously located within a full university with a "one university" concept, and location in one of the largest cities in the United States.

Identifying strategically the questions that can be asked, based on the unique strengths and environment of a school of nursing, is a requisite first step. Several directions could be taken, depending on context of the particular school:

- *Conduct efficacy studies: testing models, searching for comparison groups or data sources.*
- *Develop studies across different settings on the same topic, e.g., effects of selected therapies for a specific symptom or problem.*
- *Link with existing researchers' programs of research and "add on" a question or direction, seeking additional funding to explore new but related areas. This would be efficacious for nursing studies and to add a nursing component to an interdisciplinary study.*
- *Use a model (Donabedian, 1980; Mitchell, Ferketich, & Jennings, 1998) to frame research agendas in research-based practices in which collection of baseline and outcome measures is routine; compare outcomes across different types of settings where similar patients are served.*
- *Identify areas of expertise within the faculty and take advantage of these strengths to frame questions; for example, entice a researcher with expertise in behavioral change to collaborate in a study of nursing interventions with chronically ill individuals in a range of settings.*
- *Use management information system data to conduct exploratory studies, e.g., determine viability of a study in a particular setting; conversely. Involve researchers in helping to shape the content of management information systems so that particular questions can actually be asked of the data set.*
- *Examine the research agendas of each practice individually and as a whole. Are there cross-cutting research themes, regardless of patient population served or type of service(s) rendered, that could be exploited? Examples might include function, symptom management, risk reduction, vulnerability, transitions in care settings, or organizational contexts of care.*
- *From an interdisciplinary or cross-campus perspective, identify the themes in the strong programs of research of colleagues that would lend themselves to broader research team interest: depression, stress, sleep disorders, mind–body relationships, health disparities, illness response, and so on. These are areas in which adding on a nursing question would be efficacious and of likely interest to funders.*

- *Find ways to fertilize the practice-research integration. Link researchers with clinicians to ask new questions using strategies such as planning for dialogue within and across existing research centers and/or research teams. Develop collaboratively a strategic plan for research in academic nursing practice. Examine ways to share core research-practice resources, that is, informatics. Hold think tanks with built-in plans for continuity and follow up. Look at structure within the school to achieve the best fit; an integrative organizational design model is likely to be most effective.*

—Linda H. Aiken

REFERENCES

Baernholdt, M., & Lang, N. M. (2003). Why an ICNP? Links among quality, information and policy. *International Nursing Review, 50*(2), 73–78.

Barnsteiner, J., Ford, N., & Howe, C. (1995). Research utilization in a metropolitan children's hospital. *Nursing Clinics of North America, 30*(3), 447–455.

Bowles, K. (2000). Application of the Omaha System in acute care. *Research in Nursing and Health Care, 23*(2), 93–105.

Brooten, D., Kumar, S., Brown, L. P., Butts, P., Finkler, S. A., Bakewell-Sachs, S., et al. (1986). A randomized clinical trial of early hospital discharge and home follow-up of very low birthweight infants. *New England Journal of Medicine, 315,* 934–939.

Brown, L. A., Meier, Spatz, Zukowsky, & Spitzer, A. (1996). Use of human milk for low birthweight infants. *Online Journal of Knowledge Synthesis for Nursing, 3,* 1–9.

Brown, M. A. (2001). Academic faculty practice: Enrichment through synergism. *Applied Nursing Research, 14*(10), 56–61.

Coenen, A., Marek, K. D., & Lundeen, S. P. (1996). Using nursing diagnoses to explain utilization in a community nursing center. *Research in Nursing & Health, 19,* 441–445.

Colling, J. (1993, March 3). *Future gerontological nursing initiatives.* Unpublished Report to Dean N. Lang. Philadelphia: University of Pennsylvania School of Nursing.

Dansky, K. H., Palmer, L., Shea, D., & Bowles, K. H. (2001). Cost analysis of telehomecare. *Telemedicine Journal and e-Health, 7*(3), 225–232.

Deshefy-Longi, T., Swartz, M. K., & Grey, M. (2002). Establishing a practice-based research network of advanced practice registered nurses in Southern New England. *Nursing Outlook, 50*(3), 127–132.

Donabedian, A. (1980). *Exploration in quality assessment and monitoring, Vol. I: The definition of quality and approaches to its assessment.* Ann Arbor, MI: Health Administration Press.

Evans, L. K. (2001, November 8). *Penn Nursing Network: Summary Report to the Dean* (unpublished). Philadelphia: University of Pennsylvania School of Nursing.

Evans, L. K., & Yurkow, J. (1999). Balanced Budget Act of 1997 impact on a nurse-managed academic nursing practice for frail elders. *Nursing Economics, 17*(5), 280–282, 279.

Evans, L. K., Swan, B. A., & Lang, N. E. (2003). Evaluation of the Penn Macy Initiative to Advance Academic Nursing Practice. *Journal of Professional Nursing, 19*(1), 8–16.

Fagin, C. (1986). Institutionalizing faculty practice. *Nursing Outlook, 34*(3), 140–144.

Fagin, C. M. (2000). Executive leadership: Improving nursing practice, education and research. In C. M. Fagin (Ed.), *Essays on nursing leadership* (pp. 61–75). New York: Springer.

Gennaro, S., Fehder, W., Nuamah, I. F., Campbell, D. E., & Douglas, S. D. (1997). Caregiving to very low birthweight infants: A model of stress and immune response. *Brain, Behavior, and Immunity, 11*(3), 201–215.

Gennaro, S., Fehder, W., & York, R. (1997). Weight, nutrition, and immune status in postpartal women. *Nursing Research, 46,* 20–25.

Glancy, J., & Sochalski, J. (1999, November). *Patient characteristics, functional outcomes, and service utilization of an outpatient geriatric rehabilitation program.* Paper presented at the 52nd Annual Scientific Meeting of the Gerontological Society of America, San Francisco.

Grey, M. (1999). Why faculty must practice: The integration of practice, research, policy and pedagogy. In *Putting it all together: Proceedings of the AACN 1997 and 1998 Faculty Practice Conferences* (pp. 17–30). Washington, DC: American Association of Colleges of Nursing.

Grey, M., Lipman, T., & Cameron, M. (1997). Coping behaviors at diagnosis and in adjustment one year later in children with diabetes. *Nursing Research, 46*(6), 312–317.

Grey, M., & Walker, P. H. (1998). Practice-based research networks for nursing. *Nursing Outlook, 46,* 125–129.

Houldin, A. D., Jacobsen, B., & Lowery, B. (1996). Self-blame and adjustment to breast cancer. *Oncology Nursing Forum, 23*(1), 75–79.

Jenkins, M. (2002, April 12). Outcomes routinely documented using an electronic patient record in primary care. *Proceedings of the 28th National Organization of Nurse Practitioner Faculties Annual Meeting,* Minneapolis, MN.

Joint Task Force on Primary Care Pilot Programs (July 30, 1993). *Proposal from the Joint Task Force of the School of Medicine and the School of Nursing on Primary Care Pilot Programs.* Philadelphia: Author.

Jones, E. G., & Van Ort, S. (2001). Facilitating scholarship among clinical faculty. *Journal of Professional Nursing, 17*(3), 141–146.

Kagan, S. H., Chalian, A. A., Goldberg, A. N., Rontal, M. L., Weinstein, G. S., et al. (2002). Impact of age on clinical care pathway length of stay after complex head and neck resection. *Head & Neck, 24*(6), 545–548.

Kurlowicz, L. H. (2001). Benefits of psychiatric consultation-liaison nurse interventions for older hospitalized patients and their nurses. *Archives of Psychiatric Nursing, 15*(2), 53–61.

Lang, N. M. (1995). *Nursing data systems: The emerging framework.* Washington, DC: American Nurses Association.

Lang, N.M., Jenkins, M., Evans, L. K., & Matthews, D. (1996). Administrative, financial, and clinical data for an academic nursing practice: A case study of the University of Pennsylvania. In *The Power of Nursing Faculty Practice,* (pp. 79–100). Washington, DC: American Associate of Colleges of Nursing.

Lang, N. M., Evans, L. K., & Swan, B. E. (2002). Penn Macy Initiative to Advance Academic Nursing Practice. *Journal of Professional Nursing, 18*(2), 63–69.

Macnee, C. L. (1999). Integrating teaching, research and practice in a nurse-managed clinic. *Nurse Educator, 24*(3), 25–28.

Marek, K. D. (1997). Measuring the effectiveness of nursing care. *Outcomes Management for Nursing Practice, 1*(1), 8–12.

Marek, K. D., Jenkins, M., Westra, B. L., & McGinley, A. (1998). Implementation of a clinical information system in nurse-managed care. *Canadian Journal of Nursing Research, 30*(1), 37–44.

Mayhew, P. A. (1994). Academic practice collaboration for nursing research. *Medsurg Nursing, 3*(3), 230–231.

McCorkle, R., Strumpf, N. E., Nuamah, I. F., Adler, D. C., Cooley, M. E., et al. (2000). A specialized home care intervention improves survival among older post-surgical cancer patients. *Journal of the American Geriatrics Society, 48*(12), 1707–1713.

Medoff-Cooper, B., McGrath, J. M., & Bilker, W. (2000). Nutritive sucking and neurobehavioral development in preterm infants from 34 weeks PCA to term. *MCN: The American Journal of Maternal Child Nursing, 25*(2), 64–70.

Mitchell, P., Ferketich, S., & Jennings, B. (1998). Quality health outcomes model. *Image: Journal of Nursing Scholarship, 30*(11), 43–46.

Naylor, M., Brooten, D., Jones, R., Lavizzo-Mourey, R., Mezey, M., et al. (1994). Comprehensive discharge planning for hospitalized elderly: A randomized clinical trial. *Annals of Internal Medicine, 120*, 999–1006.

Naylor, M. D., Bowles, K. H., & Brooten, D. (2000). Patient problems and advanced practice nurse interventions during transitional care. *Public Health Nursing, 17*(20), 94–102.

Naylor, M. D., & Buhler-Wilkerson, K. (1999). Creating community-based care for the new millennium. *Nursing Outlook, 47*(3), 120–127.

O'Sullivan, A., & Jacobsen, B. (1992). A randomized trial of a health care program for first time adolescent mothers and their infants. *Nursing Research, 41*(4), 210–215.

Richmond, T. S., Kauder, D., & Schwab, C. W. (1998). A prospective study of predictors of disability at 3 months after non-central nervous system trauma. *Journal of Trauma, 44*(4), 635–643.

Sawyer, M. J., Alexander, I. M., Gordon, L., Juszczak, L. J., & Gillis, C. (2000). A critical review of current nursing faculty practice. *Journal of American Academy of Nurse Practitioners, 12*(12), 511–516.

Sochalski, J. A. (2001). Outcomes of a nurse-managed geriatric day hospital (Abstract). *Gerontologist, 41*(Special Issue), 51.

Stringer, M. (1998). Personal costs associated with high-risk prenatal care attendance. *Journal of Health Care Poor Underserved, 9*(3), 222–235.

Strumpf, N., & Evans, L. (1988). Physical restraint of the hospitalized elderly: Perceptions of patients and nurses. *Nursing Research, 37*, 132–137.

Taylor, D., & Marion, L. (2000). Innovative practice models: Uniting advanced nursing practice and education, In A. Hamric, J. Spross & C. Hanson (Eds.), *Advanced nursing practice: An integrative approach* (pp. 795–831). Philadelphia: Saunders.

University of Pennsylvania School of Nursing (1993, revised 9/21). *Long-range Plan through the year 2000.* Philadelphia: Author.

University of Pennsylvania School of Nursing (February 27, 1995). *School of Nursing Network and Penn Health System.* Presentation to Penn Health System Implementation Group. Philadelphia: Author.

Zachariah, R., & Lundeen, S. P. (1997). Research and practice in an academic community nursing center. *Image: Journal of Nursing Scholarship, 29*(30), 255–260.

Chapter 10

Establishing an Evidence Base in Academic Practice: The Role of the Clinician-Educator Faculty

Jane H. Barnsteiner, Lenore H. Kurlowicz, Terri H. Lipman, Diane L. Spatz, and Marilyn Stringer

Nursing is a practice discipline, thus, expert clinicians are vital to the tripartite mission of the University of Pennsylvania School of Nursing (UPSON). UPSON has a long and rich tradition for creating and sustaining environments in which clinical expertise is valued. Similarly, the scholarly approach to solving patient care challenges is valued in the clinical settings that UPSON operates and/or with which the school is affiliated (see Chapter 9). For more than 25 years, UPSON has been a leader in academic nursing practice among schools of nursing in research-intensive universities. A major visible component of this leadership comes from the Clinician Educator faculty.

One of the major academic faculty appointment options at the University of Pennsylvania is the clinician educator position (see also Chapter 5).

Clinician educators (CE) are members of the standing faculty who are actively engaged in practice; a proportion of the CE's total appointment is committed to a clinical agency or other practice setting. CEs enjoy the same rights and privileges as do tenured faculty save for voting on matters of tenure. This means that the CE is eligible for sabbatical leaves and participation on school and university committees and may hold administrative posts such as division chair or associate dean. Clinician educator faculty serve in teaching and leadership roles in the UPSON as undergraduate course directors and directors of graduate programs. Within the University, they serve on key task forces and committees, including the university faculty senate.

The most common arrangement is for the CE to be employed by the university, with the clinical agency "buying out" a portion of the person's appointment. A CE may have as much as 100% or as little as 20% of an appointment with the clinical agency. The Hospital of the University of Pennsylvania (HUP) and the Children's Hospital of Philadelphia (CHOP) are just two of the partnerships and alliances that offer a rich environment in which the CE can integrate the research, education and practice mission of the School of Nursing.

The success of the CE role is based on the *interrelatedness* of practice, education and research, and the *integratedness* of CEs into their respective clinical settings. The interrelatedness stems from a common basis that is rooted in a clinical phenomenon or situation, with practice, education, and research related to the topic informing and transforming each other. The extent to which this is effective relates to the degree to which of the faculty members who are functioning as CEs are integrated with both the school and the clinical institution. Rather than role strain, the potential exists for a rich synergistic exchange among practice, teaching, and research activities in both settings. In optimal situations, the curriculum is enhanced, clinically relevant faculty research is generated, community connections are established and maintained, and patients and families receive evidence-based care. It is a role that clearly closes gaps between nursing education and nursing service.

As an example, at CHOP there are four CE faculty members. Three of them are in advanced practice nursing (APN) roles. They are doctorally prepared APNs whose approach to practice is different from the traditional APN practice. They frame all of their clinical experiences through the lens of research, bringing a heightened sense of inquiry to the care of patients and to generating research questions to improve patient care. A purposeful integration of education, research, and clinical care helps to advance the science of nursing, shape the structure and quality of health care, and provide a sense of continuity in patient care and student teaching. The fourth CE at CHOP, the principle author of this chapter, serves as the director of nursing practice and research for the institution, thus, providing leadership for developing and sustaining an evidence-based practice environment (Barnsteiner & Prevost, 2002; Barnsteiner, 1996).

A hallmark of the CE role is leading and facilitating the cycle of clinical practice-research-education-clinical practice, and assuring that it is based on evidence. The four examples in this chapter illustrate how CE faculty operationalize this cycle and, thus, integrate an evidence base into their academic practice, improve the care of patients and families in the process, and enhance the education of students. The first two examples describe the work of CEs with appointments at HUP, while the last two describe the work of CEs who hold clinical appointments at CHOP.

The PALS Program[1]

Within an academic setting, one essential requirement for the CE role is the intentional linkage between a school of nursing and a clinical setting—in this case, UPSON and HUP. For the role to be successful, support is needed from both environments, with the mutual goal of bringing together novice undergraduate and graduate nursing students with clinical experts from the university medical center. The CE is in an ideal position to identify areas in which students and clinical experts share complementary agendas although their strengths differ. An example of a bridging initiative is the implementation of the student-led Philadelphia Alliance Labor Support (PALS) program in the maternity center at HUP.

PALS is a volunteer "doula" program staffed by lay persons whose goal is to enable nursing students to provide comfort and support to laboring women and their families. A doula is a professionally trained, nonmedical labor support attendant who provides continuous physical, emotional, spiritual, and advocacy support to women during labor and birth. Numerous randomized control studies have shown that a doula's presence during labor contributes to improved birth outcomes (Langer, Campero, Garcia, & Reynoso, 1986; Madi, Sandall, Bennett, & MacLeod, 1999; Wolman, Hofmeyr, Nikodem, Chalmers, & Kramer, 1993). The labor and delivery staff at HUP had identified that some patients were unaccompanied during their

---

[1]Marilyn Stringer, PhD, CRNP, RDMS—Assistant Professor of Women's Health Nursing

labor and delivery experience and needed the additional support that could be provided by a doula, but that there was no doula program in place. Although the PALS program had been successful in establishing an effective doula program, the group had limited experience in negotiating entry into a large, complex medical system. Simply stated, the PALS program needed access to a clinical site to provide this service.

The CE provided the link or bridge between the student-led group and the clinical experts in labor and delivery with a common goal of improving the support for laboring women. She did this in several ways. First, the CE was key to facilitating forums for dialogue between colleagues from nursing, medicine, and legal affairs to assist in the successful entry of the PALS program. Second, she provided evidence from the literature (see earlier text) of improved birth outcomes to support this change of practice. Third, she fostered dialogue concerning the implementation and evaluation plan for the PALS program. The successful execution of these forums led to the PALS program's becoming a valued volunteer resource available at HUP to laboring women from throughout the community.

The importance of this alliance for both groups is demonstrated in the following example of a socially vulnerable laboring young woman. A frightened 12-year-old presented herself to the delivery suite. She was alone, scared, and in labor. The experienced delivery staff knew that she needed someone to be with her during her delivery experience: This young adolescent could use the support of a doula. Because of the alliance between the school of nursing and HUP, the PALS program was able to provide additional comfort and support to this girl throughout her labor and delivery, with the outcome being a positive birth experience for this vulnerable preteen mother. It also provided a wonderful learning opportunity for students engaged in the program. This collaboration between the nursing students and the HUP staff promoted achievement of the complementary agendas of both groups through the provision of evidence based, quality care.

The success of the PALS project has been disseminated both locally and nationally. Locally, the student-led group has provided numerous presentations at both the university medical center and the school of nursing. The work of the student group was highlighted in a poster presentation at the medical center during Nurses Week. In addition, the PALS project was part of a panel discussion during alumni day activities that highlighted innovative student activities. Nationally, the PALS project was part of a segment for a public broadcasting network series (Sherman, 2000). The network interviewed and filmed one of the PALS members providing care to a laboring woman at HUP.

Two manuscripts describing the PALS project have been prepared for publication. Development of the manuscripts occurred as part of an undergraduate course requirement for two of the students, with the CE as teacher providing close supervision and guidance during the manuscript preparation process. The first student's manuscript, part of a senior-level scholarship assignment, provided a state of the science review and synthesis of the evidence supporting the use of doulas during labor and delivery, with the associated birth outcomes.

The second manuscript met two objectives: a student undergraduate course requirement and a quality improvement process for the hospital. For this student, developing a small data based project re: the design, implementation, and evaluation of a quality improvement project was the goal. The hospital's complementary need was to evaluate the PALS program following implementation. The student PALS member provided quality outcome data as feedback to the hospital 6 months after the implementation of the PALS program. The information was incorporated into the article on implementing an evidence-based doula program in a tertiary care center.

As indicated above, the nature of the role of the CE facilitated improved quality of patient care, and facilitated both the students' exposure to laboring women and opportunities for scholarly growth. The hospital benefited by having extended resources available to the patients under their care, and by being able to offer an opportunity for individual nurses to be part of a scholarly activity.

Geropsychiatric Psychiatric Consultation-Liaison Nurse[2]

At HUP, the CE provides psychiatric nursing consultation as a *GeroPsychiatric Consultation-Liaison Nurse* (GPCLN) to medical-surgical nurses and other providers caring for a complex patient population. Consisting of mostly older, acutely confused/delirious patients who are at high risk for injury while hospitalized, these patients are complex medically, psychologically, and behaviorally, and they are often placed on an increased level of nursing observation with one-to-one monitoring to assure safety. One aspect of the role of the CE is to support staff nurses and nurse managers in their systematic, individualized clinical assessments of patients using standardized instruments for delirium and/or depression. Using the patient assessment data, the CE assists the nurses with their clinical decision-

---

[2]Lenore H. Kurlowicz, PhD, RN, CS—Assistant Professor of Geropsychiatric Nursing

making regarding nursing interventions to promote safety and to make reliable judgments about the many factors that simultaneously contribute to the patients' complexities. By characterizing the individualized needs of this vulnerable group of patients and the appropriate nursing interventions, nurses are better able to make informed decisions about the need for expensive "continuous observation." Data generated from consultations with patients and their nurses have been used to establish and build on "best practices" for this patient population. From this work, an evidence-based clinical practice guideline for acute confusion/delirium and depression in older patients has been developed and disseminated (Kane & Kurlowicz, 1994; Kurlowicz, 1997).

With the CE's expertise in the care of hospitalized older adults with psychiatric and medical comorbidity and her pivotal role as an APN, scholarship and teaching are enriched for students and staff. Clinician educator faculty enjoy a unique and key position in successfully tending to the interplay between medical and psychosocial problems in hospitalized older adults, as well as to the differences in perspective among patients, families, and health care providers in this setting. The scholarly work as a CE stems from a strong personal commitment to (1) the integration of research and clinical practice in the provision of mental health care to older hospitalized adults, and (2) enhancing nursing practice for addressing mental problems in medically ill elders by bringing evidence-based knowledge to the "frontline." For example, Kurlowicz (2001) completed a study that examined the benefits of GPCLN services for older patients with delirium and/or depression, as well as for the nurses who cared for them. The findings suggest that interventions by a GPCLN contribute to quality patient outcomes in these patients. Benefits of the intervention included a reduction in distressing mental symptoms and enhanced discharge disposition. In addition, a mental health service linkage with local visiting nurse agencies for this high-risk group of patients was established. This linkage, previously nonexistent, has helped to establish a more seamless system of psychiatric nursing services for patients in recognition of their risk status for continuing mental distress post hospital discharge.

Enhancing nursing practices for complex medically and mentally ill older adults by bringing evidence-based knowledge to the bedside is the hallmark of faculty practice and speaks to the "scholarship of application" inherent in the CE's role (Boyer, 1990). Furthermore, strong collaboration with nurse researchers at the school of nursing as well as with colleagues in the departments of medicine and psychiatry makes possible the translation and application of cutting-edge knowledge to hospital care. The synergy of clinical acumen and scholarly inquiry enables the GPCLN to uniquely contribute to the education of the next generation of nurses, to the development of new knowledge, and to the search for answers to important clinical problems that ultimately may improve outcomes for vulnerable populations.

Endocrine Clinical Nurse Specialist[3]

The role of the advanced practice nurse in endocrinology at CHOP includes interviewing and examining children with a variety of endocrine disorders, educating children and families in the inpatient and outpatient settings, and coordinating the nursing care of children with endocrine disorders throughout the hospital. Questions and issues from clinical practice form the basis for a program of research, and research in turn structures the CE's practice and teaching.

The research of the *Endocrine Clinical Nurse Specialist* (ECNS) has been in two major areas that have significantly affected patient care. The first line of inquiry was initiated during dissertation research on the epidemiology of diabetes in children. Interest in this topic stemmed from multiple questions posed by parents of children with diabetes regarding possible environmental risk factors of type 1 diabetes. The ECNS developed the first diabetes registry in Philadelphia (Lipman, 1993). These data now are part of the World Health Organization's international study of the incidence of diabetes in the world. This study, which demonstrated a very high incidence of diabetes in Puerto Rican children and a low incidence in very young Black children, has prompted research in Puerto Rico and Chicago into factors that contribute to the differential development of diabetes in children of different races.

In 1993, the ECNS noted a tremendous rise in the number of new cases of children with diabetes in her practice. The second 5 years of data from the Philadelphia diabetes registry, 1990–1995, confirmed her clinical impression: There *was* an epidemic of diabetes in children throughout the city of Philadelphia in 1993 (Lipman, Chang, & Murphy, 2002). Parents of children with diabetes are often concerned about the increased risk of cardiovascular disease associated with diabetes. These concerns led her to study cardiovascular risk factors in children with diabetes (Lipman, Hayman, Fabian, 1997a, 1997b; Lipman et al., 2000a).

---

[3]Terri Lipman, RN, PhD, CRNP, FAAN—Associate Professor of Pediatric Nursing

The second program of research is in an often-neglected area of pediatric practice, the assessment of growth. The chronically ill children from the ECNS practice whose growth had been inadequately assessed prompted her research in growth in children with chronic conditions, including children with renal disease, orofacial clefting, and HIV infection (Lipman, Rezvani, Mastropieri, & Mitra, 1999; Lipman et al., 2002). This line of research is crucial for nurses working with chronically ill children, since many of the interventions for these children are based on the child's length or the growth percentile. The ENCS also noted that children were often mismeasured in primary care practices. Based on this observation, she conducted a pilot study to survey measuring practices by primary care providers. Measuring practices were found to be grossly inadequate (Lipman et al., 2000b). In 70% of primary care practices, children were being measured using incorrect techniques or inaccurate measuring devices, resulting in imprecise measurements. Growth education programs significantly improved measurement precision (Lipman et al., 2001). Data were presented at national and international meetings and the findings also received coverage by the press. In addition to affecting growth assessment on a local level, the data have impacted widely on measurement technique and precision and have served to inform parents to advocate for their children's right to accurate measurements.

As an advanced practice nurse, the ENCS works closely with nursing staff, coordinating patient care conferences and giving in-service education to new orientees and to experienced staff. Raising the level of professional practice is an important component of her role. She has coauthored articles with staff nurses (Lipman, Difazio, Meers, & Thompson, 1989a, 1989b) and edited a special edition of a journal with articles authored by nine nurse practitioners in the endocrine division at CHOP (Deatrick & Lipman, 2000).

In her role as a standing faculty member at the university, the integration of practice and teaching is core. Noting that new graduate nurses were inadequately prepared to care for children with diabetes led her to study the diabetes knowledge of new nurses. Their knowledge was shown to be deficient (Lipman & Mahon, 1999). The data from this study formed the foundation for revisions that were made to the diabetes content in the undergraduate nursing curriculum. Vignettes of clinical practice always structure her teaching. Precepting graduate students in the clinical setting afford the students the ability to learn by example.

Being both a doctorally prepared APN and a faculty member places this CE in a position to influence greatly the practice of staff nurses, nurse managers, school nurses, advanced practice nurses, undergraduate and graduate nursing students. Bringing research to the clinical site and clinical practice to the university is a model of the continuity of care and clinical scholarship envisioned for shaping health care for the future.

Clinical Nurse Specialist for Lactation[4]

Serving as a CE at Penn and clinical nurse specialist for lactation at CHOP provides a unique opportunity for clinical scholarship and research. In this position, research, education, and clinical practice are intertwined on a daily basis. The position of clinical nurse specialist for lactation at CHOP has allowed for the translation of research based protocols to be implemented directly into practice in the clinical arena. This work was supported by a grant, Breastfeeding Services for Low Birth Weight Infants (RO1-NR-03881). Increasing lactation services throughout CHOP and, in particular, improving research-based lactation services in the newborn infant center (NIC), a neonatal intensive care unit, were identified as goals in the strategic plan for the NIC.

The first step in the process of providing evidence-based lactation services was to identify the strengths and opportunities for improvement. First order priorities were (1) increasing staff knowledge regarding basic breastfeeding concepts, (2) developing standards, policies and procedures related to breastfeeding and use of human milk, and (3) procedural issues surrounding the storage and handling of human milk.

In her joint role, the *clinical nurse specialist for lactation* (CNS-L) is able to draw on her teaching experiences at the school of nursing and apply them in her role as clinical nurse specialist. Basic nurse education in the NIC was provided through inservice presentations held around the clock to maximize the number of nurses who could attend. Key content areas that are important to be addressed in a neonatal intensive care setting include milk storage and handling and successful breastfeeding techniques for vulnerable infants.

A breastfeeding resource nurse (BRN) course was also established. This course was modeled after a similar course taught to undergraduate students in the school of nursing. The BRN course is a 16-hour 2-day course that gives nurses a full overview of breastfeeding and lactation, as well as specific information related to the infants who are cared for at CHOP. The BRN

---

[4]Diane Spatz, RN, PhD—Assistant Professor of Health Care of Women

course began as a NIC initiative but has now been expanded to the entire hospital. The goal is to provide each nursing unit throughout the hospital with at least one nurse trained as a BRN. The course is offered twice a year, and, to date, more than 100 nurses have been trained as BRNs. The BRN not only has the benefit of enhancing the staff's knowledge base, but the BRN also becomes a resource person for the patient care unit. The model has been positively received and the improved support for breastfeeding has been particularly evident in the NIC.

A hospitalwide interdisciplinary breastfeeding committee was also established. Meetings with the nurse manager of each unit assisted in garnering support for the committee. This method generated enthusiasm for staff participation in the committee and support for improvement of lactation services throughout the hospital. The committee, which meets monthly, developed nursing standards and procedures, patient education materials, and identified research opportunities while providing an liaison between lactation services and the individual nursing units.

Two areas in which the CE provided leadership to improve care are illustrated here. First, breastfeeding mothers and their families require much support and education, especially when their infant is hospitalized. Leading the interdisciplinary breastfeeding committee, the CE assisted members in designing solutions to improve services. A breastfeeding teaching plan was developed that is available to be downloaded from the hospital intranet, making it available 24 hours a day. The plan is specific enough in detail that even a novice educator, with the support of the unit based BRNs, could walk a breastfeeding mother through the basics of pumping, breast milk handling and storage, positioning and latch-on, test weights, and community resources. On a daily basis, the nursing staff are more confident in their ability to provide appropriate breastfeeding education. A binder with comprehensive education materials is located on every unit for use by staff or to copy to breastfeeding mothers for their use.

A second problem that was addressed related to breast-milk management throughout the hospital. A formalized mechanism was needed for the labeling, storage, and handling of human milk that would provide consistency among all areas. A quality improvement team identified the priority areas for action. Given space and economic constraints, it was not feasible for CHOP to build a milk bank; therefore, an alternative solution was necessary. Standardized labels were developed for both pumped milk and for prepared, fortified milk. These labels are now available in all pump rooms and nourishment stations in nursing units throughout the hospital. In addition, a breast-milk-management team leader was identified for each nursing unit. Team leaders are responsible for ensuring that breast milk is properly labeled and stored in their units. Daily tracking is documented, and team leaders can immediately address any problems with their fellow staff members. These changes resulted in immediate improvement in handling and storage through a method that was effective for staff nurses and reflective of spatial and economic constraints.

Creating a breastfeeding and human milk research-intensive environment is a broader goal. The first step has been enhancing knowledge bases and addressing procedural issues. The nursing standard on breastfeeding and the policy on milk handling and storage, which are evidence-based, are in place. Evidence-based policies on the use of the breast pump, skin-to-skin care, and test weights have been developed and implemented. Because of the partnership between CHOP and the school of nursing, nursing students have participated in these changes. For example, two students developed a self-learning module for breastfeeding the preterm infant and an additional student team developed a breastfeeding-learning module for use throughout the hospital.

The unique role of combined clinical nurse specialist, educator, and researcher allows all 3 role components to flourish. One of the biggest challenges in supporting breastfeeding in vulnerable populations is the lack of health care provider knowledge about appropriate care. The CE role facilitates the effective translation of current research into practice, the provision of staff support and education, and the generation of new research ideas.

COMMON THEMES IN CLINICIAN EDUCATOR PRACTICE

The preceding faculty examples are representative of dozens of examples that are descriptive of their peers. As is so clearly evident, the stories of the APNs that are described above share several commonalities. Clinician educator faculty

(1) Possess a strong clinical knowledge base and a passion for improving the care of their respective patient populations;

(2) Not only value evidence as a basis for practice, but generate it, disseminate it, teach from it, and use it when interacting with other health care professionals;

(3) Effect patient-care improvements and organizational change.; and

(4) Enrich the educational experience of students.

Each of the clinician educator faculty descriptions applies the components of Boyer's (1990) definition of scholarship. More specifically, Boyer expanded the traditional concept of scholarship, identifying four components relevant in today's health care environment:

- *Scholarship of Discovery:* the generation of new knowledge
- *Scholarship of Integration:* the establishment of connections across disciplines
- *Scholarship of Teaching:* the transformation of knowledge and creating new scholars
- *Scholarship of Application:* engagement, an agenda that benefits society.

Faculty in research-intensive universities are engaged in all aspects of scholarship, but it is this latter category that distinguishes the CE from scholars pursuing more traditional forms. The nature of the CE role is to simultaneously generate new knowledge with an eye to the realities of clinical practice, and concurrently to establish evidence bases for that practice and for the education of tomorrow's practitioners. Employing clinical expertise as a basis for all professional activities, the CE is able to astutely identify practical issues that need attention, establish effective partnerships for tackling these issues, and incorporate the latest evidence in developing strategies for addressing them, and thus achieving significant improvements in patient care and organizational performance. While the role is challenging, clinician educator faculty value the opportunities inherent in concurrently improving practice, teaching, and research in both academic and clinical settings.

REFERENCES

Barnsteiner, J., & Prevost, S. (2002). How to implement evidence-based practice: some tried and true pointers. *Reflections on Nursing Leadership, 28*(2), 18–21.

Barnsteiner, J. (1996). Research-based practice. *Nursing Administration Quarterly, 20*(4), 52–58.

Boyer, E. L. (1990). *Scholarship reconsidered: Priorities of the professoriate.* Princeton, NJ: The Carnegie Foundation for the Advancement of Teaching.

Deatrick, J. A., & Lipman, T. H. (2000). Nurse practitioners and improved access to care for children with chronic conditions and their families. *Nurse Practitioner Forum, 1*(5).

Kane, A. M., & Kurlowicz, L. H. (1994). Enhancing the postoperative care of acutely confused older adults. *MED/SURG Nursing, 3,* 453–458.

Kurlowicz, L. H. (1997). Nursing standard of practice protocol: Depression in elderly patients. *Geriatric Nursing, 18,* 192–199.

Kurlowicz, L. H. (2001). Benefits of psychiatric consultation-liaison nurse interventions for older hospitalized patients and their nurses. *Archives of Psychiatric Nursing, 15,* 53–61.

Langer, A., Campero, L., Garcia, C., & Reynoso, S. (1998). Effects of psychosocial support during labour and childbirth on breast feeding, medical interventions, and mothers' well-being in a Mexican public hospital: A randomised clinical trial. *British Journal Obstetrics Gynaecology, 105,* 1056–1063.

Lipman, T. H. (1993). The epidemiology of Type I diabetes in children 0–14 years of age in Philadelphia. *Diabetes Care, 16,* 922–925.

Lipman, T. H., Deatrick, J. A., Treston, C. S., Lischner, H. W., Logan, J., et al. (2002). Assessment of growth and immunologic function in HIV-infected and exposed children. *JANAC, 31,* 37–45.

Lipman, T. H., Chang, Y., & Murphy, K. M. (2002). The epidemiology of type 1 diabetes in children in Philadelphia 1990–1994: Evidence of an epidemic. *Diabetes Care, 25,* 1969–1975.

Lipman, T. H., DiFazio, D. A., Meers, R. A., & Thompson, R. L. (1989a). A developmental approach to diabetes in children. Part I—Birth through preschool. *American Journal of Maternal Child Nursing (MCN), 14,* 255–259.

Lipman, T. H., DiFazio, D. A., Meers, R. A., & Thompson, R. L. (1989b). A developmental approach to diabetes in children: Part II - School age through adolescence. *American Journal of Maternal Child Nursing (MCN), 14,* 330–332.

Lipman, T. H., Hayman, L. L., & Fabian, C. V. (1997a). Risk factors for cardiovascular disease in children with type I diabetes (Part I). *Journal of Pediatric Nursing, 12,* 265–272.

Lipman, T. H., Hayman, L. L., & Fabian, C. V. (1997b). Risk factors for cardiovascular disease in children with type I diabetes (Part II). *Journal of Pediatric Nursing, 12,* 318–321,

Lipman, T. H., Hayman, L. L., Fabian, C. V., DiFazio, D. A., Hale, P. M., et al. (2000a). Assessment of risk factors for cardiovascular disease in children with Type I diabetes. *Nursing Research, 49,* 160–165.

Lipman, T. H., Hench, K., Logan, J. D., DiFazio, D. A., Hale, P. M., et al. (2000b). Assessment of growth by primary health care providers. *Journal of Pediatric Health Care, 14,* 166–171.

Lipman, T. H., Hench, K. D., Benyi, T., Clow, C., Delaune, J., et al. (2001). An intervention program significantly improves the precision of linear growth measurement in primary care practices. *Program and Abstracts of the 83rd Annual Meeting of the Endocrine Society,* 1891.

Lipman, T. H., & Mahon, M. M. (1999). Nurses' knowledge of diabetes. *Journal of Nursing Education, 38,* 92–95.

Lipman, T. H., Rezvani, I., Mitra, A., & Mastropieri, C. (1999). Assessment of stature in children with orofacial clefting. *American Journal of Maternal Child Nursing, 24,* 252–256, 1999.

Madi, B. C., Sandall, J., Bennett, R., & MacLeod, C. (1999). Effects of female relative support in labor: A randomized controlled trial. *Birth, 26,* 4–8.

Sherman, L. (Producer). (fall 2000). Birth Day: Philadelphia Alliance Labor Support. Discovery Channel.

Wolman, W. L., Chalmers, B., Hofmeyr, J., & Nikodem, V. C. (1993). Postpartum depression and companionship in the clinical birth environment: A randomized controlled study. *American Journal Obstetrics Gynecology, 168,* 1388–1393.

Chapter 11

Community–Academic Partnerships

Margaret M. Cotroneo, Joseph Purnell, Marina C. Barnett, and Danielle C. Martin

The need for an efficient and adequate health care delivery system remains at the forefront of health concerns (Institute of Medicine, 1996; Powell & Wessen, 1999; Institute of Medicine, 2001). Once again, communities are being looked to as promising settings and as potential resources for improving the system of care. Communities are facing a broad range of conditions that require a more comprehensive view of health and illness. Asthma, cardiovascular disease, hypertension, lead poisoning, HIV-AIDS, diabetes, violence, and a range of quality-of-life indicators such as smoking cessation are cases in point where a broad view of health and illness is required and where results can more effectively be achieved with community-based strategies (Olds et al., 1997; Lasker, 1997; Edelman, 1998). Complementary attention to prevention and to behavioral, familial, social, and environmental life in the communities where these problems abound is required. Progress in prevention depends on education and research in community-based population-focused health care delivery. The development, implementation, and management of community models, however, will require leadership that is capable of working effectively in and with communities to find new ways of providing services, educating students, and participating in research.

Nurses have a long history of developing successful community partnerships and health programs. Historically, nurses have managed programs and provided care to elderly, poor, and rural populations. They are generally educated to use more preventive and health-promoting interventions, to counsel and communicate with patients more frequently, and to take advantage of health education, community resources, and behavioral interventions to manage disease and disability. These are precisely the skills that are needed in a health care system that values continuous and comprehensive engagement with patients and their families to preserve health (Pew Health Professional Commission, 1998). Public health nursing programs and community nursing organizations are long-standing examples of this work (see Chapters 2 & 12). In this chapter, potential responses to health care challenges are explored and analyzed through their application in an academic nursing center owned and operated by the University of Pennsylvania School of Nursing (UPSON).

COMMUNITY–ACADEMIC PARTNERSHIPS: PRINCIPLES AND STRATEGIES

Experts have produced dozens of questions and some solutions to the problem of how to involve communities in the health care system. The literature suggests that it is important to know and understand the resources and barriers to partnership from the perspective of community participants (Kretzmann & McKnight, 1993; Sullivan & Kelly, 2001). Communities are often viewed by academic institutions in terms of their liabilities, such as lack of involvement of ethnic/minorities in the health care system in general, impact of poverty, distrust, varying health beliefs, and disparities in health and quality of life. When the members of a community are seen as dynamic assets, however, it increases the possibility of mapping their relationships to the health care system, mobilizing their networks, and matching their interests with those of academic institutions. Communities are experts in their own processes and dynamics, and they can leverage their knowledge in collaborating with academic institutions (Kretzmann & McKnight, 1993; Sullivan & Kelly, 2001). Essentially, this approach incorporates elements of the shared-power perspective, in which professionals strengthen and support community capacity and self-efficacy by providing a climate, a relationship, resources, and procedural means through which people enhance their own lives. In this context, researchers and communities approach their work together as collaborative partners.

A number of experts (Kretzmann & McKnight, 1993; Freudenberg, Eng, Flay, Parcel, Rogers, & Wallerstein, 1995; Richards, 1996; Sullivan & Kelly, 2001; W.K. Kellogg Foundation, 2002) have identified the central characteristics of this partnership as:

- Community-based leadership and ownership of specific programs
- Training and utilization of community residents for leadership
- Projects tailored to a specific population and a specific setting
- Involvement of participants in planning, implementing, and evaluating proposed projects
- Use and further development of existing community resources
- Sequenced planning to address various problems in culturally sensitive, competent ways
- Interdisciplinary community practice and training opportunities for faculty and students
- Links between individual, family, community, environmental/contextual services and policy levels
- Health concerns linked to a vision for a better quality of life
- Collaborative arrangements with existing health care provider networks

Community–academic health center partnerships not only have the opportunity to benefit and enhance the health-related quality of life of communities, but they also provide considerable benefit to the academic health institution in educating health professionals for the future and in translating and transmitting knowledge to benefit and serve humanity. Indeed, the latter has traditionally been considered the civic duty of academic institutions.

Despite increasing attention to the value of community-based approaches to research and education in the health professions, community–academic partnerships face multiple barriers and problems. Specifically, while academic institutions may be willing to establish partnerships with community organizations, to many minority populations, the institution's research agenda, as applied to health, carries several negative connotations. This includes perceptions of academic institutions as being dishonest, arrogant, unfair, and exploitive. The Tuskegee Syphilis Study informs many African American community groups and individuals, and this shapes their mistrust of health-related projects that are proposed by academic institutions (Corbie-Smith, Thomas, Williams, Moody-Ayers, 1999). Communities have prior experiences of not having been consulted by academic institutions in matters that directly affected them and of culturally insensitive and incompetent interactions with students, faculty and other institutional representatives, many of whom lack training in working with communities.

On the other hand, partnering with community structures is challenging because community-based organizations may be loosely formed, and, as such, may be composed of an assemblage not necessarily conducive to collaborative decision-making among academic and community-based groups. Such structures may also make it more difficult to identify community leadership and access potential partners. Further, communities have internal conflicts and power struggles. Dialogue about projects and activities can easily be derailed. Community relational processes can be intensely circular, requiring a long-term commitment of time and resources for trust to develop. This process may be out of step with the more linear processes of academic environments.

Community–academic partnerships must acknowledge and incorporate the culture and the social context of the recipients academic institutions are trying to reach. This willingness and ability to draw on community-based values, traditions, and customs and to work with knowledgeable persons of and from the community in developing targeted interventions, communications, and other supports is one example of cultural competence (Health Services and Resources Administration [HSRA], 2001; Airhihen-buwa, 1999). Finally, partnerships with communities are dynamic and generative, grounded in the needs and aspirations of the partners and established on the strengths and resources of the partners. At the core is a long-term commitment to relationships of trust and reciprocity.

Since 1993, the authors have been working together and with community groups and organizations to develop a sustainable, mutually beneficial partnership. The formal contact exists through established community groups, while a nurse-managed health center, operated in the community UPSON's Penn Nursing Network (PNN), has provided informal contact with many community residents, giving the collaboration a continuing service presence.

NETWORKING FOR SUCCESS AND SUSTAINABILITY: CASE ILLUSTRATION

In 1993, UPSON embarked on a broad initiative to integrate its primary-care practice network, which consisted largely of faculty-led practices operating in isolation of each other. Given the emerging national primary health care agenda and the promise of health care reform, the long-term aim was to develop models of academic–community practice consistent with the school's tripartite mission of education, practice, and research. Except for isolated faculty efforts, UPSON as an entity did not have a strong community presence.

The school's initiative was made possible by a five-year grant from the Health Services and Resources Administration's Division of Nursing, continuous support from the Philadelphia-based Independence Foundation, and a community-based nursing leadership grant from the Helene Fuld Health Trust. The vehicle for this initiative was the Health Annex, a family and community academic nursing center, located in Southwest Philadelphia and serving the underserved communities of Paschall-Kingsessing. The Health Annex is a partnership between UPSON, the Philadelphia Department of Recreation, and the community of Paschall-Kingsessing (Cotroneo, Outlaw, King, & Brince, 1997a, 1997b). The initial project team from UPSON included the first author as lead faculty, a pediatric nurse practitioner/doctoral student as project coordinator, and an undergraduate nursing student and a master's level psych-mental health nursing student.

The University of Pennsylvania is located in the heart of West Philadelphia and is bordered by a number of neighborhoods, each with its own characteristic social demography, culture, and history of relationships to the university. The neighborhoods of West Philadelphia share a relationship with the university that can best be described as a "wary symbiosis." It is shaped by self-interest but not necessarily trust, with many ethical dilemmas characteristic of asymmetrical relationships. There is also a long history of trusted individuals and groups working together, however, that has helped to bridge some of the distrust.

Given that history and guided by the principle that communities are primarily relational configurations, the project team focused on the process of trust building. This process began at the ground level and consisted of four components: (1) conducting an interactive assessment of needs, strengths/assets, and key stakeholders, (2) identifying trusted and respected community consultants who were of the community, (3) networking with potential community partners, and (4) establishing a service presence in the community.

A Contextual Assessment

The project team drove through the West Philadelphia neighborhoods to take a look at the living environment—block by block—and locate community services—recreation centers, schools, churches, health centers, and so on. Using a snowballing technique in which each contact identified one or several others, a series of meetings were then set up with key community individuals, groups, and organizations already serving the community (e.g., Black Women's Health Project, Neighborhood United Against Drugs, Presbyterian Homes, Cornerstone Christian Academy, and the Myers Recreation Center Advisory Board). Advice was sought about community needs, deficits, strengths, and assets. Available demographic and health-related data were examined, following which the team returned to meet again with some of the community individuals and groups. Nursing students were involved at every step of the process.

What emerged was the identification of the neighborhood of Paschall-Kingsessing in Southwest Philadelphia as an underserved community in need of primary care services. One of the contacts, a public health nurse employed with the city health department, set up a series of meetings with the Commissioner of the Philadelphia Department of Recreation, who had a plan for integrating health care into selected city recreation centers. As a result of those meetings, together with three planned and open community meetings, the project team was expanded to include the commissioner and vice-commissioner of recreation, the president of the community advisory board of the Myers Recreation Center, and the project's two community consultants. In a two-year period, this partnership resulted in newly designed and renovated space for a family and community health center in a building "annexed" to the city recreation department in the Paschall-Kingsessing community. A 10-year memorandum of understanding defined the partnership.

Use of Community Consultants

In the partnership model, entry to the community is through identified community leaders and trusted professionals working in the community. Through networking with individuals and groups, a consultant was identified who became part of the team, coaching members to navigate through some of the so-called mine fields that potentially exist in under-resourced communities. Among her key recommendations were face-to-face meetings with local politicians of every persuasion who had a stake in the community to engage their support. Another key recommendation involved planned, open community meetings to lay out the agenda in detail and provide an opportunity for community residents to get their questions answered and their concerns addressed. The quality of relationships in a community is shaped by communitarian (collective) as opposed to individual values (Airhihenbuwa, 1999; McKinlay & Marceau, 2000). Transparency, truth telling, power, and reciprocity are among the most important communitarian values, and learning their meaning in real terms requires direct face-to-face relating to community residents. The wisdom of a community—the meanings inherent in the experience and voice of its citizens—is only transmitted in this process of engaging with communitarian values and beliefs. Students and faculty who go into a community focused on individual tasks miss this level of understanding.

On the advice of the consultant, face-to-face meetings were also scheduled with community-based organizations, local physicians, and the proximate city health department clinics to clarify aims, areas of overlap in services, and potential collaborations. Meetings with key local businesses such as the neighborhood pharmacy, the vision center, food markets, communities of faith, and the community newspaper helped the team gain an insider understanding of community life. Through meetings with these stakeholders, suggestions came forward from the community about who might best serve on a community advisory board, and the group of community advisors was expanded to include the second author of this chapter. This approach to community participation in the proposed project eventually resulted in an advisory board for the Health Annex that actually represented the community's interests.

In the networking process, strong resistance among some individuals in the community was expressed. These individuals felt that resources that might flow into the community through the city's recreation department should not go to a university-sponsored project. They were vocal and politically active in their attempts to exercise control over the outcome. In the end, however, the project had enough support from trusted community groups and individuals to move it forward. It also had the support of the local politicians who had been brought on board from the beginning. From the design and furnishing of the Health Annex to the hiring of personnel, every effort was made to reflect the community, whose residents are primarily of African descent. Community residents were hired as outreach workers, personnel who were persons of color were recruited to staff and manage the center, an African American-owned construction company managed the renovations, an architect who had a special commitment to community health centers designed the space, and the works of African-American artists and craftspersons decorated the interior. In trying to hold to a standard of cultural competence and quality of care, mistakes in judgment were made along the way, but the community advisors helped the team avoid the most serious breeches of trust.

Communities are complex webs of people, located in a particular time and place, shaped by relationships, interdependence, mutual interests, and patterns of interaction (Richards, 1996). The building of academic–community relationships requires investments of trust, fairness, reciprocal care, clear expectations, and attention to obligations and promises. Partnership is possible only when there is leadership from the community and when the academic health center is willing to make the long-term commitment. Service to the community is a concrete manifestation of trust. Establishing a service presence in the community even before the Health Annex opened its doors was one of the most critical decisions the team made, and it was made on the good counsel of the community advisors who were also residents of the community. While the team was generally sensitive to the broader issues of race and ethnicity, these advisors helped UPSON develop a deeper understanding of the dynamics of relationship embedded in race; for example, race and ethnicity are often secondary to the overall quality and trustworthiness of the relationship but racism is an ever-present reality to be addressed. From the service delivery perspective, issues of class emerged more often than did issues of race in both black-black relationships and black-white relationships, yet racism and class and the expectations attached to them receive little attention when providers are trained for practice in community-based health systems.

Nursing students took the leadership in establishing a service presence in the community during all of these negotiations. From 1993–1995, the students demonstrated UPSON's values and commitment through mentoring projects for youth at the recreation center; offering health education programs (e.g., dating relationships, smoking, safe sex, conflict resolution, safety on the playground, gun violence), organizing a community health fair, participating in community meetings and community outreach activities, and linking the recreation center, their base of operation, with university resources and with other students. They were the service presence of UPSON in a community that had had little or no experience with nursing providers. Community residents got to know them personally and asked for them specifically. The students made a difference, and they knew it, demonstrating yet again the close relationship between nursing values and communitarian values.

Creating Opportunities for Meaningful Collaboration

Creating opportunities for collaboration through planned activities and projects tests the trust base of the relationship and works out imbalances in power and resources. The decision-making process around opening the Health Annex exposed the fragmentation that existed in the community itself. In 1996, community residents who wanted a voice in matters that affected them organized themselves into a coalition of groups called the Southwest Community Action Coalition (SWAC). SWAC is a trusted community resource that includes 30 community-based organizations, of which the Health Annex is one. It is a part of a broader network of 200 community organizations and churches, the Southwest Community Alliance. SWAC members cooperate with each other in community development activities. SWAC activities include outreach to block captains, churches, recreation centers, and health centers. SWAC and the Alliance function as internal community governance structures, safeguarding and promoting the community's interests and coordinating the planning process for community development activities and proposed projects in the community.

The advantage of having an alliance such as SWAC is that it facilitates service and research projects, improves access to community resources and assets, and provides partnering institutions like a university with continuity of relationship to community leadership. The disadvantage occurs when personal agendas override the communal agenda, resulting in the alliance functioning more as gatekeeper than facilitator. It is usually a real or perceived injustice that triggers the reactivity, which in the past would have derailed any progressive ideas from being seeded. With greater internal organization, however, community leadership is able to refocus issues toward more positive outcomes.

From the outset, the Health Annex had two aims to its mission. The first was to deliver high quality comprehensive, culturally competent primary health care. The second was to engage with the community in community development activities. Delivering collaborative health services in a community-based setting carries with it some responsibility for community development. Community development is a process of working in collaboration with a community to assess needs and desires and to address these needs through the use of local talent, resources, and management (Lassiter, 1992). The Family Festival and Community Health Fair became the first major collaboration that addressed both aims.

The Health Annex community outreach worker, also a resident of the community, took responsibility for the planning and implementation (including fundraising) of this annual event sponsored by the community for the community. With access to Penn students from the dental, nursing, and medical schools and the Bridging the Gaps Community Health Internship Program, together with donations from managed care companies with whom the Health Annex had contracts, participation by local and city-wide organizations, SWAC, churches, city health and recreation departments, and donations from local businesses, the Festival brings almost every facet of the community together for a day of health promotion, health screenings, games for children, entertainment, and giveaways of health-related items. Attendance for this event has grown to 3,000 community residents. The community has visibility and a positive profile beyond its geographic boundaries. Political candidates understand the importance of showing their support by their attendance.

Central to making this kind of collaboration possible is the staff position of the community outreach worker, dedicated to both health-related activities and to community development activities. When the Health Annex opened, so pressing were the socioeconomic needs of the residents that primary health care and prevention were not even listed among the community's top ten priorities. The link between health and quality of life had to be made. Most of the outreach worker's time is spent outside the physical space of the Health Annex, linking with community-based organizations and keeping health care on the community's list of priorities. The Health Annex always has a seat at the table of any decisions that affect the community and reliable feedback on issues that concern the community.

Outreach is the thread that weaves the biopsychosocial tapestry of service delivery, yet it often goes unrecognized as one among other services in the academic health center that employs the outreach worker. The University of Pennsylvania, however, recently instituted an annual service of excellence award ceremony to recognize employees' service to the university community. As a member of the academic community, the Health Annex community-outreach worker was one of those honorees.

Further Evolutions of Community–Academic Partnerships

Through collaborative projects like the Family Festival, the community consultant model evolved into a mentorship model. Community residents and organizations and Penn faculty and students mentor each other in a reciprocal process. This happens most effectively when shared knowledge is the motivation for the arrangement. With funding from the Jessie Ball duPont Foundation, the Health Annex partnered with Neighborhood United Against Drugs (NUAD) to design and implement a men's health outreach initiative. The project leader is a men's health assistant who is a community resident trained and supervised jointly by NUAD and the Health Annex staff. Baccalaureate and master's level Penn students learn public health skills by working with the outreach worker and health assistant in service delivery, compiling epidemiologic data about men's health and sociodemographic data about men in the community, designing and implementing population-focused health education/health promotion activities, and facilitating focus groups. NUAD and the Health Annex share the grant funding. Outcomes data are collected and shared by both organizations. The project itself is linked to larger university faith-based and school-based initiatives targeting prevention and health disparities through the university's Center for Community Partnerships. In this way, local projects are nested in larger projects that address national health policy agendas. This ability to link with broader policy initiatives is one of the effectiveness tests for local projects.

Community-partnered research, a sequenced planning process for jointly designed, implemented and evaluated research projects is another evolution of the partnership model (Minkler, 2000; Israel, Schulz, Parker, & Becker, 1998). Increasingly, community-based or community-partnered research is being recognized as an essential element of reducing racial and ethnic disparities in health-related outcomes (North American Primary Care Research Group [NAPCRG], 1998; Sullivan & Kelly, 2001). In November 2001, the National Institute for Nursing Research (NINR) and the National Center on Minority Health and Health Disparities (NCMHD) convened a state-of-the-science meeting called Community-Partnered Interventions in Nursing Research to Reduce Health Disparities. The participants identified components of successful interventions—for example, trust, long-term commitment, partnerships, shared power, mutual appreciation of needs and priorities, inclusion of a service component, and implementation of findings into policy. The group identified health promotion, chronic conditions, and environmental and cultural considerations as promising areas for research (NINR, 2001).

A community-based research approach is a form of collaborative inquiry that utilizes a team approach to identify and understand the broader social and environmental context of health behaviors and risks. The partnership extends to all phases of the research process and provides a built-in mechanism for dissemination of research findings. Health care and health care research are viewed in a social context; institutions must refocus their objective to involve communities rather than individuals in the research enterprise. By involving communities, institutions can broaden the research agenda from solely recruitment to the full range of decision-making relevant to research: planning, recruitment, data collection, interpretation, and dissemination of results. Involving communities in research requires effective formal and informal relationships between minority communities and academic institutions. Central to this approach is the ability of the community to understand the process and the methodology of the research.

As stated before, a level of mistrust often is associated with research conducted in the African-American community. Much of this mistrust can be attributed to miscommunication in the delineation of the research process itself. UPSON contracted with a researcher whom the community identified to serve as a liaison to explain the project's technical vernacular in meaningful ways that could be understood by the community. This ability to utilize the existing resources of the community is another aspect of the shared power perspective discussed earlier.

Over the past year, the authors, together with colleagues from the University of Pennsylvania School of Medicine, Temple University School of Social Administration, and two community-based organizations, have studied the use of complementary and alternative therapies or medicine (CAM) in a population of low-income African Americans in local communities. To reach this population, the study team used a culturally sensitive method (modified focused group interviews) to collect data, in conjunction with culturally sensitive survey instruments designed in partnership with residents from the community from which the sample was drawn. This partnership resulted in recruitment of 72 subjects and the development of instruments and protocols for a larger study of CAM use in local African American communities.

The sequenced planning process for the project involved the following steps:

- An idea is generated
- A planning group of potential community partners and Penn research team is convened
- Community partners report to constituent community groups
- A small community consultant group is formed
- The community consultant group and the Penn research team reconvene as the project team

The planning process has also worked in the reverse when community partners approached a Penn research team to respond to an RFP on smoking cessation, maternal child health, or children's mental health. The sequenced planning process is critical for several reasons. Promising more than can be delivered by either group erodes trust. It is better to decline if mutual interests cannot be met. Population-focused projects require teams committed to the project from start to finish. In spite of the good intentions of committed individuals, a real team on one side must be balanced by a real team on the other. The budget process must be transparent for partners to weigh the benefits and burdens of partnering in material and financial terms.

The great advantage of community-partnered research is that community partners often have resources and strengths in grant writing, recruitment, data collection, and dissemination of findings that have been underused because academic health centers have not incorporated the community's knowledge and experience in the planning process. A sequenced planning process among the partners is the sine qua non of all successful community–academic partnerships.

By providing subjects in the community with a place at the research table and a tangible return for their participation, investigators can begin to erode the long-held perception that research is conducted more for the benefit of the academic investigators than for the benefit of the communities involved in the study. In community-partnered research, investigators must be sufficiently open to consider the perspective of community residents and flexible enough to implement the community's recommendations. Perhaps the most crucial aspect of establishing community-partnered research is making sure that the community's goal for the research is met. In the CAM study, for example, pilot data from focus-group interviews with African Americans suggested that a worthwhile product from researching CAM use among African-American groups would be data that educated the community about CAM, informed physician education programs, and facilitated the formation of culturally competent systems of care. Thus, this project was linked to a larger project to train researchers to partner with minority communities in conducting research.

Community-Based Nursing Leadership Curriculum

In July 1998, the School of Nursing of the University of Pennsylvania was funded by the Helene Fuld Health Trust, HSBC Trustee, to design and develop a community-based nursing leadership curriculum aimed at creating and integrating community-based models into our emerging health care system (Salmon et al., 1999). This master's curriculum focused on expertise in four curricular areas: (1) leadership for community-based health systems development, (2) health-related community development, (3) population-focused health interventions, and (4) program development and administration. The project itself was designed in phases, which included an in-depth review of the literatures relating to the four curricular areas. Internal and external advisory groups were formed to guide the project throughout its development. Two nationally known experts in the areas of public health and community health leadership advised the project staff throughout the duration of the project. The project identified areas in which providers need to build their knowledge base if they are going to work effectively with communities, including:

1. Defining the nature and characteristics of a community.
2. Identifying key determinants of healthy communities.
3. Forming a partnership with a community.
4. Demonstrating community assessment strategies and methods.
5. Analyzing a community's formal and informal organization.
6. Identifying and mapping community assets.
7. Assisting communities in building their competence and self-determination.
8. Interacting with communities in culturally sensitive and appropriate ways.

The project staff believed that that the structural foundations of any community-based nursing leadership curriculum must allow nurses to work within their own sector while at the same time linking up with other professionals in other sectors of the health care delivery system. The ability to create structures that honor both the individual and the common health enterprise is at the heart of community-based care. Collaborative curricular arrangements are the most amenable structures to support that effort.

THE FUTURE IS NOW

In a 1998 policy statement, NAPCRG summarized the process of establishing community-academic partnerships: "Full partnership takes time to establish and requires maturation of trust; development of vision, confidence, skills and knowledge; and a gradual shifting of balance and perspective through genuine, respectful dialogue. It follows, then, that certain skills and qualities are advantageous in this continuous process of negotiation and compromise" (p. 5).

The tools, skills, and knowledge for community-academic partnerships have received considerable attention from the knowledge areas of family medicine, public health, public health nursing, social work, primary care, and psychiatric-mental health nursing, but they have not made their way into general curricula. Instead, they have tended to operate on the periphery of the educational system much as prevention remains on the periphery of the health care system.

Dedicated efforts continue to be made at the University of Pennsylvania to build service-learning electives or incorporate service-learning projects into existing courses. Service learning is defined as "structured learning experience that combines community service with explicit learning objectives, preparation and reflection" (Seifer, 1998, p. 274). These individual efforts, involving undergraduates across all 12 of Penn's schools, are highly rated both by students and the faculty who teach them. They are largely isolated from each other, however, and, thus, the knowledge that has been accumulated cannot be leveraged into broader perspectives and disseminated in ways that would benefit populations and influence policy. Service learning in the community–academic partnership model would call for working with communities to identify their priorities. Each student group could then build on the work of a preceding student group to address those priorities from a continuous rather than from a fragmented approach.

A service presence in the community, linked to education and research and modeled after the community-academic partnership models like the one described here, offers promise for the future of America's health care delivery system. Academic nursing centers such as the Health Annex are preparing community-based nursing leadership and seeding ideas for curricular innovations that capture the minds and hearts of the brightest and the best students (Cotroneo, Kurlowicz, Outlaw, Burgess, & Evans, 2001). Partnership models are expensive to maintain, however, without cost-based reimbursement for the service entity itself, as many nurse-managed centers have learned (Hansen-Turton & Kinsey, 2001). Movements underway to leverage the resources of these centers through strategic alliances and then to link their agendas to the broader policy agenda may be effective in the long run (see Chapters 12 & 13). Leadership—trained and experienced in community-based health care delivery—must be a priority for academic health centers if community–academic partnerships are to realize their potential to shape the health care culture. Leadership development itself, however, must be a partnership with communities.

REFERENCES

Airhihenbuwa, C. O. (1999). Of culture and multiverse: Renouncing 'the universal truth' in health. *Journal of Health Education, 30*(5), 267–273.

Corbie-Smith, G., Thomas, S. B., Williams, M. V., & Moody-Ayers, S. (1999). Attitudes and beliefs of African Americans toward participation in medical research. *Journal of General Internal Medicine, 14,* 537–546.

Cotroneo, M., Outlaw, F., King, J., & Brince, J. (1997a). Integrated primary health care: Opportunities for psychiatric-mental health nursing in a community-based, nurse-managed primary care practice. *Journal of Psychosocial Nursing, 35*(10), 21–27.

Cotroneo, M., Outlaw, F., King, J., & Brince, J. (1997b). Advanced-practice psychiatric-mental health nursing in a community-based nurse-managed primary care practice. *Journal of Psychosocial Nursing, 35*(11), 18–25.

Cotroneo, M., Kurlowicz, L., Outlaw, F. H., Burgess, A. W., & Evans, L. K. (2001). Psychiatric-mental health nursing at the interface: Revisioning education for the specialty. *Issues in Mental Health Nursing, 22*(5), 549–69

Edelman, M. W. (1998). Keynote address. *Journal of Urban Health, 75,* 623–633.

Freudenberg, N., Eng, E., Flay, B., Parcel, G., Rogers, T., et al. (1995). Strengthening individual and community capacity to prevent disease and promote health: In search of relevant theories and principles. *Health Education Quarterly, 22*(3), 290–306.

Hansen-Turton, T., & Kinsey, K. (2001). The quest for self-sustainability: Nurse-managed health centers meeting the policy challenge. *Policy, Politics, & Nursing Practice, 2*(4), 304–309.

Health Resources and Services Administration (2001). *Cultural competence works.* Rockville, MD: U.S. Department of Health and Human Services, Bureau of Primary Health Care. Available at www:hrsa.gov/financeMC/ftp/cultural-competence.pdf. (Accessed on November 1, 2002.)

Israel, B. A., Schulz, A. J., Parker, E. A., & Becker, A. B. (1998). Review of community-based research: Assessing partnership approaches to improve public health. *Annual Review of Public Health, 19,* 173–202.

Institute of Medicine (1996). *Primary care: America's health in a new era.* Washington, DC: National Academy Press.

Institute of Medicine (2001). *Crossing the quality chasm: A new health system for the 21st century.* Washington, DC: National Academy Press.

Kaye, G., & Wolff, T. (Eds.) (1997). *From the ground up: A workbook on coalition building and community development,* 2nd ed. Amherst, MA: AHEC/Community Partners.

Kretzmann, J., & McKnight, J. (1993). *Building communities from the inside out: A path toward finding and mobilizing community assets.* Evanston, IL: Northwestern University Institute for Policy Research.

Lasker, R. D. (1997). *Medicine and public health: The power of collaboration.* New York: The New York Academy of Medicine.

Lassiter, P. G. (1992). A community development perspective for rural nursing. *Family and Community Health, 14,* 29–39.

McKinlay, J. B., & Marceau, L. D. (2000). Public health matters: To boldly go . . . *American Journal of Public Health, 90*(1), 25–33.

Minkler, M (2000). Using participatory action research to build healthy communities. *Public Health Reports, 115,* 191–197.

National Institute for Nursing Research (2001). Community-partnered interventions in nursing research to reduce health disparities. Available on www.nih.gov/ninr/news-info/pubs/interventions.pdf. Accessed September 2, 2002.

North American Primary Care Research Group (November, 1998). *Responsible research with communities: Participatory research in primary care: NAPCRG policy statement.* Available on www.NAPCRG.org/rrpolicy.html (Accessed August 18, 2002.)

Olds, D. L., Eckenrode, J., Henderson Jr., C. R., Kitzman, H., Powers, J., et al. (1997). Long term effects of home visitation on maternal life course and child abuse and neglect. Fifteen year followup of a randomized trial. *Journal of the American Medical Association, 278*(8), 637–643.

Pew Health Professions Commission, The Center for the Health Professions (1998). *Recreating health professional practice for new century: The fourth report of the Pew Health Professions Commission.* San Francisco: University of California.

Powell, F. D., & Wessen, A. F. (Eds.) (1999). *Health care systems in transition.* Thousand Oaks, CA: Sage Publications.

Richards, R. (Ed.) (1996). *Building partnerships: Educating health professionals for the communities they serve.* San Francisco: CA: Jossey-Bass.

Saleebey, D. (Ed.) (1997). *The strengths perspective in social work practice.* Boston, MA: Addison-Wesley Longman.

Salmon, M., Cotroneo, M., Couch-Jones, M. A., Mark, H. D., Mood, L. H., et al. (1999). *The community-based nursing leadership curriculum: Planning for the future health of communities.* Report to the Helene Fuld Health Trust, HSBC Trustee. Philadelphia: University of Pennsylvania School of Nursing.

Seifer, S. D. (1998). Service-learning: Community-campus partnerships for health professions education. *Academic Medicine, 73*(3), 273–277.

Sullivan, M., & Kelly, J. G. (Eds.) (2001). *Collaborative research: University and community partnership.* Washington, DC: American Public Health Association.

W. K. Kellogg Foundation (2002). Community participation can improve America's public health systems. Available on www.wkkf.org/Pubs/Health/TurningPoint/Pub3713.pdf (Accessed November 1, 2002.)

Chapter 12

Building Alliances:
A Survival Strategy

Lois K. Evans, Joanne M. Pohl, and Nancy L. Rothman

Exemplars by Tine Hansen-Turton and Margaret Grey

cademic practice affords schools of nursing the greatest opportunity
to advance the science of nursing through the integration of the
tripartite mission of education, research, and clinical care (Lang,
Evans, & Swan, 2002; Evans, Jenkins, & Buhler-Wilkerson, 2003). Academic practice is often achieved through contractual faculty practice arrangements, strong affiliations with health entities or systems, and/or
school-owned enterprises (see also Chapters 3 & 5). Even with best intentions, however, full mission integration remains an elusive goal for most
(see Chapter 9). Faculty engaged in practice often express a sense of
isolation, role overload, and lack of appreciation from administrators for
the value and nature of their work (Walker, 1995; Rudy, 2001). Affiliations
that have little control over practice models, data systems, and quality
complicate the ability to achieve mission goals. Further, practices in which
schools of nursing hold full equity can strain the infrastructures of institutions that have primarily had educational and research missions at their

core. In addition, many of these innovative equity practice models have suffered from lack of access to mainstream reimbursement mechanisms, making sustainability a critical challenge.

Recent recognition by schools of nursing of the "power in partnerships" has led to the establishment of a number of networks, collaboratives, consortia, or other alliances that hold promise for solving some of these problems. This chapter describes in detail with two of those experiences. It focuses on the benefits, risks, and lessons to be learned through the efforts of these alliances to enhance growth and sustainability of academic nursing centers and other academic practices, promote collaborative research and community-based education, and have an impact on public policy.

BACKGROUND

For many historical and current reasons, practice remains the least developed arm of the tripartite mission in most schools of nursing (see Chapter 2; Evans et al., 2003). While its importance in a practice discipline like nursing is a given, provision of clinical care is more often marginalized in universities, taking a back seat to research and educational goals. Further, small patient panels served by individual faculty members or by school-owned and operated practice entities are by themselves insufficient to support research, provide full educational experiences for students at all levels, or wield the power needed in local, state and national arenas to access funding sources. Without adequate data, numbers, and income, recognition and long-term sustainability of practice entities remain but dreams. Schools have attempted innovative collaborations for academic practice development, such as the University of Iowa's Nursing Collaboratory partnership (Dreher, Everett, & Hartwig, 2001), University of Texas–Houston's partnership with its own university to provide student and employee health services (Mackey & McNiel, 1997), and Temple University's unique collaboration with community members to mount research programs that are of interest and benefit to, and comanaged by, community and faculty partners (Rothman, Lourie, & Gaughan, 2002). Companion chapters in Part II of this book address several strategic resources to support academic practice, such as infrastructure, advisement, information systems, and so on. This chapter focuses on a particular strategy: that of building alliances, including peer networks, partnerships, collaborations and consortia, to bring sustainability, credibility and positive outcomes to academic practice.

Principles of Partnering and Collaboration

Alliances are associations of organizations formed to serve a mutual purpose, such as increased collective power or enhanced access to scarce resources, which is less effectively or efficiently accomplished by one organization alone (Zuckerman, Kaluzny, & Ricketts, 1995). A common phenomenon in the corporate business world, alliances are increasingly seen in health care. Many of the business benefits and costs of alliances summarized by Zuckerman and colleagues also apply to academic nursing practice. For example, academic nursing practice alliances can provide the opportunity to gain resources, share risks, share costs of technology development, gain influence over a domain, gain group synergy, and strengthen competitive position (Zuckerman et al., p. 4). Conversely, such alliances may also result in loss of resources (especially when the partners are unequal); loss of autonomy and control; conflict over domain, goals and methods; and delays in solutions due to complexities of coordination (Zuckerman et al.). The commitment model rather than a control model best illustrates these types of partnerships. "Such a model underscores the importance of designing and communicating common purposes, developing realistic expectations, and clearly framing the domain, scope, and activities of an alliance" (Zuckerman et al., p. 11). Alliance formation can be described in life-cycle terms as selection or courtship, engagement, setting up housekeeping, learning to collaborate, and changing within (Kanter, 1994). Constant vigilance and nurturing is required to maintain strategic alliances over time. The hallmarks of successful alliances as explicated by Zuckerman et al. (1995, pp. 5, 12–13) are similar to principles of good partnerships espoused by others (Sebastian, Davis, & Chappell, 1998); namely, appropriate partner(s) selection; shared objectives; explicit boundaries, rules, and agreements; commitment of time, energy and resources; mutual trust, cooperation and understanding; and mutual risk-sharing and learning within the alliance.

Alliances in Support of Academic Nursing Practice

Over the past decade, several examples of strategic alliance building have arisen among schools of nursing and other partners to enhance achievement of the tripartite mission through academic practice. The Penn Macy Initiative to Advance Academic Nursing Practice (with emphasis on enhancing mission integration in all types of academic practice models) and its outcomes are described in Chapter 13. Penn Macy Fellows have expressed interest in the development of a research alliance, although efforts are still very much in the early developmental stages of "courtship" and "engagement" (Kanter, 1994). Meanwhile, the Agency for Healthcare Research and Quality (AHRQ) has funded APRNet, a network to support collaborative research among advanced practice nurses in community settings on the east coast (see Exemplar A; Deshefy-Longi, T., Swartz, M., & Grey, M, 2002) and also the Midwest Regional Nursing Centers Consortium (AHRQ, 2002) to develop a similar research network among its member nursing centers. Because the alliances discussed in this chapter involve community-based academic nursing centers, a brief description of the nursing center model and two representative alliances is provided as background for the analysis of common barriers, challenges and lessons learned.

ACADEMIC NURSING CENTER HISTORY

Nursing centers have been variously defined, but most people in the field agree that they are entities that are managed by nurses and provide directly-accessible nursing care to clients—individuals, families, and communities (Frenn, Lundeen, Martin, Riesch, & Wilson, 1996; Matherlee, 1999; Task Force, 1987). Increasingly called on to serve as safety-net providers for the underserved, yet out of the funding mainstream, nursing centers exist on the precipice: at least half do not survive (Vincent, Oakley, Pohl, & Walker, 2000]. While there is no single registry for nursing centers, recent estimates confirm that as many as 250 still exist (Watson, 1996; Clear, Starbecker, & Kelly, 1999), the bulk of them associated with or owned by schools of nursing. As a group, these academic nursing centers suffer from invisibility in their universities and in the health care industry, lack of ability to tap into common health care funding streams, a tendency to operate in isolation, poor or nonexistent data to support outcomes, and small numbers of clients and services that limit student experiences, research opportunities and bargaining power (Anderko & Uscian, 2001; Frenn et al., 1996; Mackey, Adams, & McNiel, 1994; Vincent et al., 2000).

The current state of affairs is no accident. Following a decade-long emphasis on faculty practice associated with burgeoning advanced practice educational programs, community-based academic nursing centers emerged as a promising model for schools of nursing to embrace. Far from being a new concept (Lang, 1983; Frenn et al., 1996; Task Force, 1987; see also Chapter 2), the academic nursing center was nonetheless heralded as an entity that would permit the continuous practice of faculty while serving as a living laboratory, both to demonstrate the outcomes of nursing-focused services and also to educate students at all levels. Early nursing centers were as likely as not to have served the middle class (Barger & Rosenfeld, 1993). A 1980s program of the Division of Nursing, Bureau of Health Professions, Health Resources Services Administration (HRSA), however, targeted the creation of nursing centers to care for the underserved as one method of preparing the nursing workforce for community-based care. This program appears to have influenced the more recent emphasis on serving vulnerable populations (Hansen-Turton & Kinsey, 2001; Clear et al., 1999; Matherlee, 1999). The relatively ready availability of capital afforded by HRSA for initiating community nursing centers made such an endeavor possible for many more schools of nursing. Between 1986 and 1998, the HRSA division supported the development of 90 of these centers (Clear et al., 1999). Once created, each center was expected to become self-sustaining within three to five years. All over the United States, faculty in isolated schools of nursing began struggling, de novo, to create these nursing delivery models. Not until 2001 was there any effort on the part of HRSA Division of Nursing to bring grantees together to share both successes and barriers, to learn from one other, or to develop a common database (Anderko & Kinion, 2001).

As part of the grant requirement, schools of nursing have historically made significant financial investments in these centers; 10 years ago schools reported supporting 50% of the costs (Barger & Rosenfeld, 1993), although more recent data indicate that the level is now commonly at 25% or less (Vonderheid et al., 2002). Some deans have begun to question the wisdom of such investment since these centers have historically failed at about a 50% rate, most often owing to lack of financial sustainability and/or solid business practices (Vincent et al., 2000). Further, as there was no explicit research focus for these Division of Nursing-supported academic nursing centers, data requested in grant reports were limited primarily to the involvement of students. Thus, there was neither the incentive nor funding support to develop client databases for supporting outcomes research or documenting the extent and quality of care provided by these innovative safety net providers.

Beginning in the early 1980s, the National League for Nursing (NLN) had provided an organization called the Council for Nursing Centers as a place for nursing center leaders to share struggles and successes. Later, its Community Health Accreditation Program (1995) published *Standards of Excellence for Community Nursing Centers*. Without the NLN's continuing financial or operational support, however, the Council for Nursing Center's interest group had all but disbanded by the mid-1990s. Other attempts at the national level to convene interested parties generated great enthusiasm but little follow-through in terms of organizational development (Anderko & Uscion, 2001).

While each individual academic nursing center served only a limited number of clients, evidence amassed over time that these models of care delivery were well received by their clientele and that they produced powerful outcomes in the communities they served, for instance, fewer emergency room visits, higher immunizations rates, and shorter lengths of hospital stay (Hansen-Turton & Kinsey, 2001; Jenkins & Torrisi, 1995). The opportunity for these models to inform policy on a broader level was thwarted, however, by the constant threat of sheer survival. Academic nursing centers found common primary care reimbursement models to be unduly restrictive or inaccessible because of state or insurer policies. As much as anything, these sustainability issues motivated schools with centers to create, in the decade of the 1990s, collaborative affiliations that would increase the size of the client base, give focus to a health-policy agenda, provide for the sharing of resources and best practices, and give new life to this nursing delivery model. Centers survived in the interim by creating patchworks of short-term funding, while seeking a longer-term solution. Several private foundations, including the Robert Wood Johnson Foundation, the W.K. Kellogg Foundation, and the Philadelphia-based Independence Foundation, have funded nursing center projects. Some have also supported the development of collaborative alliances such as the Philadelphia-based Regional Nursing Centers Consortium, which is now known as the National Nursing Centers Consortium (NNCC) (see Exemplar B), and the Michigan Academic Consortium (MAC); these alliances were initiated in 1996 and 1998, respectively. While there are others (for example, in 2001, the Midwest Nursing Centers Consortium [MNCC@uwm.edu] was formalized), the experiences from the NNCC and the MAC provide documentation for this analysis of alliances supporting academic nursing practices and centers. For each, a brief description follows, as well as a discussion of barriers, challenges, and successes.

National Nursing Centers Consortium

As was stated earlier, this alliance was originally formalized as the Regional Nursing Centers Consortium. The impetus was a common interest in supporting a growing number of community-based nursing centers in the Delaware Valley (Pennsylvania, Delaware, and New Jersey). Funds remaining from a national conference on nursing centers, organized by LaSalle and Temple Universities and supported by the Independence Foundation, made the consortium possible. Together, the high level of regional interest and availability of funds provided the investment needed to capitalize on a set of mutual needs that has led to mutual reliability, trust, cooperation, and understanding among member nursing centers.

During this same period, the Independence Foundation convened regular meetings of the holders of the four Philadelphia-area Independence-endowed chairs in nursing—at LaSalle University, Community College of Philadelphia, Temple University, and the University of Pennsylvania—in support of community health education and service needs of the region. One outcome was a white paper (Evans, Kinsey, Rothman, & Tagliarini, 1997) that addressed and proposed solutions for the health needs of Philadelphia, which was presented to local funding agencies and policy makers at a special meeting. Having named nursing centers as one of its philanthropic priority areas, the Independence Foundation had been assisting nurse-managed health care centers in the region by grants supporting operating costs associated with serving the uninsured and the underinsured. Since each of the schools with an Independence chair had an academic nursing center, the chair holders also contributed both formal and informal leadership to the alliance development.

During its incubation phase, the NNCC was housed in the New Beginnings program of a Philadelphia-based community development organization, Resources for Human Development. In accordance with its bylaws, the consortium established a governing board with elected representatives from member centers/schools and hired a staff, including an executive director with extensive public policy expertise. Mission, vision, and goals (see Exemplar B) were made real by a facilitated strategic planning process. The governing board met monthly and the entire membership met at least annually. Multiple committees and task forces provided ample opportunity for member centers and interested parties to be involved.

Collaboration vs. competition. The mutual need for an alliance was continually fueled by the constant threat of survival experienced by each nursing center member. The risk-taking associated with sharing between and among centers was reframed as a means for mutual gain, thus lessening the vulnerability that each center faced alone. Collaboration among schools of nursing, many of which competed regularly for students, clinical laboratory sites, and research grants and lived within competitive health-system environments, represented a change in tradition. Still, communication between and among schools was often hampered by differing missions, philosophies, goals, and institutional contexts as well as differing models for care delivery that were held dear by each entity. The special languages and paradigms of each school—often a stumbling block—had to be learned and understood. Finally, it was not always easy to convince school and university administrators that interdependence among the schools, including developing grant proposals together rather than competitively, was not only a win-win but also a necessity. Such collaborative grant writing was most difficult the first time, especially since the application was unsuccessful. That experience, however, facilitated the development of a process that continues to be refined and has now resulted in many instances of successful funding. The "conspiracy of silence" between academic nursing programs had, thus, been shattered. Frank discussion about when it is acceptable to compete and when it is necessary to collaborate now occurs. Real dialogue (Senge, 1990), literally "around the table," has facilitated this process. Four discrete areas in which the collaboration has been especially fruitful—implementing clinical information systems, applying for grants, designing quality management programs, and influencing policy—are described in the following paragraphs.

Implementing Clinical Information Systems. In the NNCC, member centers had the need for information technology and networks that would allow them and the consortium to represent the whole as greater than the sum of each part to health policy makers and third-party payers. This was perhaps the greatest impetus for collaboration, as it was easy to see the opportunity for mutual gain. Different centers were each creating databases in order to have information for operations and quality management. One project, based at the University of Pennsylvania and funded by the Independence Foundation, initiated a collaborative process among area nursing centers to develop a set of common data elements and definitions that would facilitate data sharing with the shared aim of enhancing research and influencing policy (Marek, Jenkins, Westra, & McGinley, 1998; see also Chapter 8). As the NNCC matured organizationally, this project was transferred to it; with much shared effort and continuing support from the Independence Foundation; a state-of-the-art electronic information system is currently being introduced in selected member centers.

Applying for Grants. Once the alliance was established, there were new opportunities to respond to requests for proposals—and in a timely fashion. Also, the aggregation of the centers increased greatly the numbers of providers and clients served, making any application of greater interest to potential funders. For example, the NNCC now coordinates and manages several community nursing leadership programs in education, health education, and primary prevention for its member centers. One such example began with Lead Awareness: North Philly Style (Rothman et al., 2002), a NINR-funded, community-driven, community-based research project at the Department of Nursing, College of Allied Health Professions of Temple University. This program demonstrably increased the numbers of children tested and lowered blood lead levels in experimental versus control census tracts. The protocol served as a best-practice model that was leveraged in three NNCC proposals now funded by the Environmental Protection Agency: Lead Safe Babies, Asthma Safe Kids and Real Action Directed to Improving Children's health And Lifestyle (RADICAL). Several NNCC member nursing centers' in Philadelphia participate in these projects, each sharing in the resultant funding and also benefiting from the local neighborhood good will engendered by such programs.

Demonstrating quality. Common databases are advantageous for demonstrating outcomes of the member centers collectively. The tighter the collaboration, the greater the similarity between languages and paradigms, thus allowing best practices to be shared easily across academic nursing centers. The NNCC developed document called Quality Management Program Guideline for member centers in 2001 that will facilitate centers' work in this regard (Evans, 2002; www.nationalnursingcenters.com).

Influencing policy. Further, data from an aggregated group of clients and providers have proved to be of great interest to policy makers, for example, efforts to gain prescriptive privileges for advanced practice nurses in Pennsylvania. It has been increasingly clear that influencing federal health policy would be essential for the alliance to meet its mission, which is "to strengthen the capacity, growth and development of nurse-managed health centers to provide quality health care services to vulnerable populations and eliminate health disparities in underserved communities." Thus, with membership in the consortium already extending beyond the Delaware Valley, movement from a regional to a national orientation was a natural next step. In 2002, and with full board and center member support, the consortium moved physically from its original sponsor, Resources for Human Development, to the Philadelphia Health Management Corporation where it became a subsidiary 501c3 organization with its new name, the National Nursing Centers Consortium. From this vantage point, the NNCC has worked successfully with the Bureau of Primary Care at HRSA to include nursing centers in the planned expansion of community health centers.

Exemplar B by Tine Hansen-Turton, Executive Director of the NNCC, describes the many programs and accomplishments of this alliance over its first five years. As with all alliances, NNCC in its new national forum is challenged to continue to focus and refocus on long-term needs of its membership, to clearly understand the motivation and expectations of member centers, to identify mutual performance measures, and to foster trust and balance in commitment and power of its membership (Zuckerman et al., 1995).

Michigan Academic Consortium

This consortium had its roots in a new collaboration involving faculty from several schools of nursing who shared a mutual need for funds to address advanced practice nursing educational and reimbursement issues in Michigan and nationally (Pohl, Bostrom, Talarczak, & Cavanagh, 2001). Effort was first initiated when schools from two universities came together collectively to seek funding for their academic nursing centers that were each addressing the needs of very low-income populations. Although this initial effort was unsuccessful, the membership was expanded and support was then sought from a foundation (W.K. Kellogg Foundation) to achieve very broad and far reaching goals that included the tripartite missions of each of the universities. This consortium developed as do many in business as described by Zuckerman and colleagues (1995). There was a set of mutual needs, a willingness to share risks and costs as well as knowledge, and a desire to reach common objectives. The consortium members are four state universities in Michigan and their schools/colleges of nursing: Grand Valley State University (Grand Rapids), Michigan State University (East Lansing), the University of Michigan (Ann Arbor), and Wayne State University (Detroit). In addition, a fifth partner, the Michigan Public Health Institute (MPHI), provides a fiduciary role and coordinates the evaluation process. This fifth partner, sometimes referred to as the "neutral" partner, has also been most helpful in bridging old competitions or conflicts between universities. Having this partner in the fiduciary role was also a key strategy for success. Between the four schools, a total of nine nursing centers that provided full primary care services to very diverse populations were in operation. A more complete description of the project and its history is reported elsewhere (Pohl et al., 2001). The consortium members learned early on that to be effective, survive financially, and meet the health care needs of some of the most vulnerable, collaboration to inform policy with a strong unified voice would be critical. In addition, since most of the nursing centers were small, combining databases with data on outcomes and cost of care would permit the telling of a more robust story.

Goals and structure. The consortium's overall goals were to

- Work together to educate nurse practitioners to deliver more cost-effective and community responsive primary care to unserved, underserved, and Medicaid insured clients
- Increase the availability and accessibility of high quality, appropriate, effective, cost-efficient primary care delivered by nurse practitioners (NPs) in intra- (within the nursing discipline) and interdisciplinary collaborative practices
- Increase the ability of NPs to combine humanistic, business, and scientific components of primary care to improve measurable outcomes in a managed care environment through curricula and practice delivery models
- Enhance the expertise of NPs in promoting healthy lifestyles and accessing health care resources across the life span
- Prepare NPs to deliver community responsive care
- Design strategies that would ensure long-term financial viability and integrate nursing centers with the broader health care delivery systems of the communities in which they reside
- Inform policy as it relates to advanced practice nursing and nurse managed centers.

MAC had a lead institution (University of Michigan) that housed a project director and support staff. Although this was a partnership, identifying clear leadership was important. Consistent with the advice of Zuckerman and colleagues (1995), relationships in the partnership were "fragile and characterized by change" (p. 11), yet a strong belief persevered that the schools were stronger as a group than they were separately. Ongoing evaluation of satisfaction with the partnership revealed across all four years of the project a very high level of satisfaction with the leadership, the process, and the communication among all partners.

While there was one named lead institution, leadership was shared at various levels. There were multiple task forces (e.g., on education, policy, finance, evaluation), each chaired by different persons from the partner institutions. MPHI's role in assisting with the very complex evaluation process was most helpful, but the leadership for this effort came from a university. There was representation from all partner institutions on every task force and committee. A steering committee, consisting of at least two members from each of the partner institutions, met face-to-face monthly to make all decisions regarding the project. Because this involved substantial travel time, other options were considered; while some of the task forces did use teleconferencing with success, it was unanimously agreed that face-to-face contact was critical for the serious discussions and decisions that needed to be made by the steering committee.

Benefits of the alliance. Although sustainability issues and policy issues are what initially brought the members together, it became clear early on that many more benefits could be realized from the collaboration if there were willingness to share opportunities and take risks. Opportunities to share curriculum as well as details of practice operations proved to be a benefit beyond expectations. Shared modules in the subject areas of managed care, finance and business practices for advanced practice nurses, serving the underserved, cultural competence, and informing policy as advanced practice nurses were all critical products that would not have been developed without collaboration. Openly sharing curriculum materials was not initially easy. It meant taking the risk to admit gaps and needs. Once those fears were overcome, the benefit in terms of improved products demonstrated the worth of risk-taking.

One of the major successes involved informing policy and occurred early in the project. Working together, MAC and the Michigan Nurses Association gained a rules change in Medicaid reimbursement in Michigan so that all nurse practitioners, not just family or pediatric nurse practitioners, could be reimbursed for primary care services. Efforts have been continued to inform policy both at the state and national level. This was an important early lesson about the power of the alliance.

Some of the major benefits in collaboration included sharing expertise in the business of practice between the universities and various nursing centers. Since some of the nursing centers in this consortium had many more years of experience, they were able to provide support and advice to the less mature centers. The outcomes from this sharing proved to be exponential in that centers benefited more than could have been facilitated by any one school. A key strategy for financial sustainability was the development of a financial advisory committee made up of experts in business and finance as well as nursing faculty and practitioners. The work of this group brought together all of the nursing centers; the outcome was much stronger financial and business practices.

Other opportunities afforded by the consortium included exchange of student clinical placements. Although this was limited, it did occur and proved to be very successful. A major benefit was the ability to obtain quality outcome measures on key diagnoses such as asthma, hypertension, diabetes, breast and cervical cancer screening, and childhood immunizations. This was the start of developing outcome benchmarks for member centers. Cost of care in member centers was also better understood through collaboration, thus, sustainability was markedly improved with collaboration. This was partially true in that together member centers were able to bring in expertise and share the cost and the wisdom of the expert. In addition, by joining forces, better pricing on software was obtained.

Scholarship was a major opportunity offered through this consortium. Multiple paper or poster presentations (a total of 47) have been made at state, national, and international meetings. Each paper shared authorship across at least two of the four universities and often across all four universities as well as the fifth partner, MPHI. To date, there have been more than 10 papers that have either been published, are in press, or are under review.

Challenges and barriers. There was and remains to some extent a history of competition across all four universities. A major concern was whether such history of competition could be overcome to facilitate reaching a larger goal. A key lesson over the first four years was that, while the competition did not disappear, members learned to work with it and around it and to acknowledge it publicly when it interfered with progress. A common refrain used by members was, "The power of the consortium is worth it," meaning that while working together was challenging, the benefit was well worth the cost. Many would now say that to achieve success in a nursing center, collaboration is essential.

Policies at each university vary, presenting challenges. Not all of the universities had faculty practice plans; those that did, however, were able to offer advice and assistance to the others. Each university also had its own business operations procedures and infrastructure, creating some difficulty in managing all of the centers similarly. For example, the goal that every center would use the same software package for practice management and electronic medical records (EMR) to make data collection consistent was not, in the end, realistic due to the software specification requirements in place at some of the universities. Consistent with the literature (Zuckerman et al., 1995), a major challenge to collaboration was that everything seemed to take longer than anticipated. Working with various universities and their unique bureaucracies simply meant that decisions would often not be made as quickly as preferred. While individual members often grew impatient, there were no easy solutions, despite all of the advantages of technology. Perhaps the greatest challenge was selecting an EMR. Because of the state of the technology and limited resources, this decision took the longest of any in the project. In the end, a decision was made to pilot this effort at *two* centers in *one* university, pooling funds across *all* universities. Reaching consensus on the specific centers for implementing the pilot was relatively easy. While laborious and much more difficult, the decision regarding the product paled in comparison to reaching agreement on the sharing of funds! Overcoming the old notion of "what's mine is mine" was not easy, but members recognized that a major breakthrough in consortium development had been achieved on the day agreement was reached to actually give up funds to reach the overall goals.

BENEFITS, COSTS, AND LESSONS LEARNED

The trust that evolved over time between members in the two alliances enabled sharing of information and data previously held "close to the chest" (quality outcomes, financial data) and facilitated a sense of solidarity and common mission. As the previous descriptions and analyses make clear, however, all members experience both benefits and costs as well in forming alliances. These can be summarized by drawing from Zuckerman and colleagues' *Strategic Alliances* (1995).

Common Benefits

Benefits for those forming alliances include the opportunity to

- *Gain resources.* Examples include sharing cost of piloting the EMR at MAC, developing a CIS at NNCC, having access to business expertise, shared negotiations with payers and policy makers, collaborating on projects and funding opportunities, sharing clinical placements, sharing quality measures.
- *Share risks.* Likewise, sharing cost of piloting an EMR meant that no one school had to bear the full expense, yet each could learn whether it worked.
- *Share costs of technology development.* Examples include CIS and EMR development, sharing course curricula, developing common guidelines for quality management program.
- *Gain influence over a domain.* Both alliances became major spokespersons for nursing centers at the local, state, and, increasingly, national levels.

- *Gain group synergy.* Representative membership on task forces and committees and having success by using "one voice" at policy tables are examples.
- *Strategic competitive position.* The ability to compete successfully for grants, to negotiate for better rates for purchase of an EMR, and the policy efforts exemplify this benefit.

Common Costs

Alliance formation is not without costs. For the alliances described, these included

- *Loss of resources.* Giving up money to support an EMR pilot in someone else's center and perceived loss of access to funding sources (when the alliance is the grantee) are examples of these costs.
- *Loss of autonomy and control.* Having to share grants and share leadership, giving up opportunity to individually negotiate a "better deal" with payers by going with the alliance, and longstanding cultures of competition for funding and prestigious opportunities are examples.
- *Conflict over domain, goals, methods.* These were revealed through the differences in language, paradigms, and mission.
- *Delays in solving coordination problems.* In striving to reach buy-in and consensus, everything took longer.

Lessons Learned

To become a *learning organization* (Senge, 1990), two principles are imperative. First is embracing the belief that both positive and negative lessons have value. Second is that replication, regardless of the first outcome, also has value, especially when it is difficult to generalize between populations and contexts. Everyone loves to share positive outcomes, but it is equally important to share negative ones to prevent others from spinning their wheels. For both alliances described here, it was perhaps the ensuing *dialogue* that occurred as people (representing institutions) got comfortable really listening and sharing, coming to view each other as colleagues, embracing the multiple meanings presented, and accepting that such a group becomes "open to the flow of a larger intelligence" (p. 239) that finally revealed the rich benefits of alliance-building. These two alliances have demonstrated strong predispositions to develop as learning organizations, and, in that light, they offer the following summary of lessons learned:

- Everything takes longer
- There is power in numbers, and a unified voice speaks powerfully
- Survival is a strong motivator for building alliances
- Sharing resources and expertise is wonderful!
- Taking risks is very difficult, especially when it involves scarce resources (funds)
- Contributions by partners tend to be uneven, i.e., not everyone pulls the same weight
- There is some loss of autonomy
- Competition does *not* disappear
- The whole really *is* more than the sum of its parts

Future of Alliances in Support of Academic Nursing Practice

Where academic nursing programs have traditionally been competitive around recruitment of students, ownership of clinical settings, and external funding for special projects, nursing centers have helped schools to overcome this tradition. The successes of the alliances have helped schools and centers acknowledge the need to come together and confirmed the positive nature of collaborating. Only through collaborative networks and consortia has the tide begun to swing in favor of long-term sustainability of academic nursing practices. In testament to this trend, and the success of the alliances in shaping the domain, is the renewed interest of the W.K. Kellogg Foundation in supporting academic nursing center development at a national level. The lessons each alliance has learned should serve it well in its relations with each other and with the new networks and consortia that are now developing. Each of these, with similar goals of securing the success of nurse delivery models for health care, is now engaged in similar dialogue with one another to reach agreement and develop strategies that will serve the whole. Learning to dialogue openly, keeping communication open to share positive and negative outcomes, and having the big picture goal at the center are essential if the discipline—and ultimately the society—is to benefit from the lessons learned.

Exemplar A.
Advanced Practice Registered Nurses' Research Network.

Practice-based research networks (PBRNs) are a group of practices devoted principally to the care of patients but also affiliated with each other for the purpose of investigating the phenomena in clinical practice occurring in communities (Greene & Lutz, 1990). Such networks have existed in medicine for 25 years, but only recently have advanced practice nurses in primary care discovered their power for studying primary care as delivered by nurses, about which little is known (Grey & Walker, 1998). Thus, Advanced Practice Registered Nurses' Research Network (APRNet) was conceived as the first PBRN for advanced practice nurses as an approach to the rigorous study of primary care delivered by nurses.

APRNet was developed with funds from the Agency for Healthcare Research and Quality (AHRQ, grants HS11196), the Robert Wood Johnson Executive Nurse Fellows Program, and matching funds from the Yale School of Nursing. The mission of APRNet is to operate a practiced-based research network of APRN clinicians working in diverse primary-care settings throughout New England. The purpose of APRNet is to conduct and facilitate practice-based research relevant to APRN primary care practice, develop culturally competent, evidence-based practice models for APRNs, and enhance the translation of research findings into primary-care practice. The network will serve as the setting for a series of research studies designed to answer questions about advanced practice nursing in a regional primary care setting, to facilitate the development of evidence-based practice models for APRNs, and to aid in translating research findings into primary care practice (Deshefy-Longhi, Swartz, & Grey, 2002).

To establish the network, a coalition of six schools of nursing was formed (Yale, Boston College, and the University of Massachusetts at Amherst and Wooster and in Connecticut and Rhode Island). Representatives from each of these schools met to discuss the network and develop the plan for recruiting members. After approval from the Yale Human Subjects' Research Review Committee, potential members were solicited using preceptor lists from each of the schools' preceptor lists as well as membership lists of APRN organizations. Currently, APRNet has 68 members from Connecticut, Massachusetts, Rhode Island, New Hampshire, Vermont, and Maine. The majority of the members are family or adult nurse practitioners and pediatric nurse practitioners. Most work in private practices with physicians or in community based clinics. These APRNs care disproportionately for the minority populations (54%) and underinsured (60%). The majority of their patient visits are for episodic illness or care of chronic illnesses. Several research projects have been conducted or are currently in progress including a replication of the National Ambulatory Medical Care Survey (NAMCS) and a study of clinician and patient understanding of data privacy and confidentiality in primary care.

The experience of APRNet is relevant to the development of academic nursing centers as we seek to study and understand the outcomes of such practice. Academic nursing practices can ally themselves with APRNet or develop their own PBRN. If developing an independent network, the following tasks are crucial: (1) Pursue funding for the infrastructure to support the network, (2) begin by developing an age-sex registry of patients served, (3) begin to develop researchable questions, and (4) enhance linkages among academic practices. PBRNs that connect academic nursing practices have the potential for significantly advancing our understanding of nursing practice.

—Margaret Grey

Exemplar B.
National Nursing Centers Consortium

BACKGROUND

Established in 1996, the National Nursing Centers Consortium (NNCC) is the first national association of nurse-managed health centers in the United States. The vision of the NNCC is to improve the health of its communities through neighborhood-based health care services that are accessible, acceptable, and affordable. The mission is to strengthen the capacity, growth, and development of nurse-managed health centers to provide quality health care services to vulnerable populations and to eliminate health disparities in underserved communities. Its three overarching goals are to provide national leadership in identifying, tracking, and advising health care policy development; to position nurse-managed health centers as a recognized mainstream health care model; and to foster partnerships with people and groups who share common goals. NNCC comprises academic- and community-based nurse-managed health-center members, associate members, and individual members.

SERVICES

NNCC provides a wide array of services and technical assistance to its member health centers, including but not limited to business and strategic

development, health center development, program development and support, marketing and public relations, information systems and data sharing, research, public policy, staff training and conferences, information
list-serve, funding support, newsletters, and networking. The NNCC
Annual Conference is held every fall. In addition, NNCC holds leadership,
clinical, and professional continuing education meetings, training, and
seminars throughout the year. NNCC publishes the NNCC Update twice
a year. It also publishes ongoing program and policy information in
relevant journals with national distribution. Staff present at multiple
national conferences throughout the year, representing nurse-managed
health centers.

PROGRAMS

NNCC has a strong history in coordinating and managing health education and primary prevention programs for its member health centers.
Programs include, but are not limited to, Lead Safe Babies, a best-practice
in-home primary prevention program; Asthma Safe Kids, an in-home
asthma trigger prevention program for children with asthma under the
age of 18 years; Radical Youth (Real Actions Directed to Improving
Children's health And Lifestyle), a peer-to-peer environmental health
training program targeted to children from the ages of 10 to 16; the
PEW Depression Training Program, a training program for professional
nurses at all levels targeted to identify, diagnose, and, when appropriate,
treat depression in primary care settings; the Beck Fellowship, a fellowship in cognitive therapy training for advanced practice nurses; the
Cardiovascular Risk Reduction Program, a joint program with the Health
Promotion Council to identify and provide nutrition and exercise counseling to woman of risk for cardiovascular disease; and the Helene Fuld
Leadership Program, a nursing leadership program targeted to student
nurses at all levels to introduce them to community-based health care
issues and solutions in nurse-managed health centers. NNCC also manages a data-mart research network of six health centers, which recently
received a generous gift to purchase the Misys electronic medical record
(EMR) and electronic practice management (EPM) system. Finally,
NNCC offers to any member center free access to its health promotion
and primary health-care data collection software.

ACCOMPLISHMENTS

Policy

NNCC was successful in getting funding through the Centers for Medicaid and Medicare Services to conduct a nursing center demonstration project evaluating 15 nurse-managed health centers. The Senate Health, Education, Labor, and Pensions Committee included language in its October 11, 2001, report supporting passage of the Health Care Safety Net Act (S. 1533), which recognized nurse-managed health centers as essential safety-net providers and would, thus, make nurse-managed health centers eligible to receive Section 330 funding (or to be certified as FQHC look-alikes), all of which are elements critical to the sustainability of the centers.

Funding

In 2001–2002, the NNCC, through its advocacy and grant writing, was instrumental in member health centers receiving more than $2.5 million in program funds and gifts.

For more information about the NNCC please visit www.national nursingcenters.com

—*Tine Hansen-Turton*

REFERENCES

Anderko, L., & Kinion, E. (2001). Speaking with a unified voice: Recommendations for the collection of aggregated outcome data in nurse-managed centers. *Policy, Politics, & Nursing Practice, 2*(4), 295–303.

Anderko, L., & Uscian, M. (2001). Quality outcome measures at an academic rural nurse managed center: A core safety net provider. *Policy, Politics & Nursing Practice, 2*(4), 288–294.

Agency for Health Research & Quality (October 18, 2002). AHRQ awards new grants to primary care practice-based research networks. *Electronic Newsletter,* Issue #74. www.ahrq.gov (accessed October 2002).

Barger, S., & Rosenfeld, P. (1993). Models in community health care: Findings from a national study of community nursing centers. *Nursing & Health Care, 14*(8), 426–431.

Clear, J., Starbecker, M., & Kelly, D. (1999). Nursing centers and health promotion: A federal vantage point. *Family & Community Health, 21*(4), 1–14.

Community Health Accreditation Program (1995). *Standards of excellence for community nursing centers.* New York: National League for Nursing.

Deshefy-Longi, T., Swartz, M. K., & Grey, M. (2002). Establishing a practice-based research network of advanced practice registered nurses in Southern New England. *Nursing Outlook, 50*(3), 127–132.

Dreher, M., Everett, L., & Hartwig, S. (2001). The University of Iowa Nursing Collaboratory: A partnership for creative education and practice. *Journal of Professional Nursing, 17*(30), 114–120.

Evans, L. E. (2002, June). *A regional approach to quality in community-based nursing centers.* Paper presented at The American Nurses Association 2002 Biennial Convention, Philadelphia.

Evans, L. K., Jenkins, M., & Buhler-Wilkerson, K. (2003). Academic nursing practice: Implications for policy. In M. D. Mezey, D. O. McGivern, & E. Sullivan-Marx (Eds.), *Nurse practitioners: Evolution of advanced practice* (4th ed., pp. 443–470). New York: Springer.

Evans, L. K., Kinsey, K. K., Rothman, N. L., & Tagliareni, E. (1997, March). *Health care for the 21st century: Greater Philadelphia style.* White Paper prepared for the Independence Foundation, Philadelphia.

Frenn, M., Lundeen, S. P., Martin, K. S., Riesch, S. K., & Wilson, S. A. (1996). Symposium on nursing centers: Past, present and future. *Journal of Nursing Education, 35*(2), 54–62.

Greene, L. A., & Lutz, L. J. (1990). Notions about networks: Primary care practices in pursuit of improved primary care. In *Proceedings, primary care research: An agenda for the 90s.* Bethesda, MD: Agency for Health Care Policy and Research.

Grey, M., & Walker, P. H. (1998). Practice-based research networks for nursing. *Nursing Outlook, 46,* 125–129.

Hansen-Turton, T., & Kinsey, K. (2001).The quest for self-sustainability: Nurse-managed health centers meeting the policy challenge. *Policy, Politics & Nursing Practice, 2*(4), 304–309.

Jenkins, M., & Torrisi, D. L. (1995). Marketing and management: Nurse practitioners, community nursing centers, and contracting for managed care. *Journal of the American Academy of Nurse Practitioners, 7*(3), 119–124.

Kanter, R. M. (1994). Collaborative advantage: The art of alliances. *Harvard Business Review, 72,* 96–108.

Lang, N. M. (1983) Nurse-managed centers. *American Journal of Nursing, 83*(9), 1290–1293.

Lang, N., Evans, L., & Swan, B. A. (2002). Penn Macy Initiative to Advance Academic Nursing Practice. *Journal of Professional Nursing, 18*(2), 63–69.

Mackey, T. A., & McNiel, N. O. (1997). Negotiating private sector partnerships with academic nursing centers. *Nursing Economics, 15*(1), 14, 52–55.

Mackey, T. A., Adams, J., & McNiel, N. O. (1994). Nursing centers: Service as a business. *Nursing Economics, 12*(5), 275–279, 282.

Marek, K. D., Jenkins, M., Westra, B. L., & McGinley, A. (1998). Implementation of a clinical information system in nurse-managed care. *Canadian Journal of Nursing Research, 30*(1), 37–44.

Matherlee, K. (1999). *The nursing center in concept and practice: Delivery and financing issues in serving vulnerable people* (Issue Brief No. 746). Washington, DC: National Health Policy Forum.

Pohl, J. M., Bostrom, A. C., Talarczyk, G., & Cavanagh, S. (2001). Development of an academic consortium for nurse-managed primary care, *Nursing and Health Care Perspectives, 22*(6), 308–313.

Rothman, N., Lourie, R. J., & Gaughan, J. (2002). Lead awareness: North Philly style. *AJPH, 92*(5), 739–741.

Rudy, E. B. (2001). Supportive work environments for nursing faculty. *AACN Clinical Issues, 12*(3), 401–410.

Sebastian, J. G., Davis, R. R., & Chappell, H. (1998). Academia as partner in organizational change. *Nursing Administration Quarterly, 23*(1), 62–71.

Senge, P. M. (1990). *The fifth discipline: The art and practice of the learning organization.* New York: Doubleday.

Task Force to Develop Guidelines for Nurse-Managed Centers (1987). *The nursing center: Concept and design.* Kansas City, MO: American Nurses Association.

Vincent, D., Oakley, D., Pohl, J., & Walker, D. S. (2000). Survival of nurse-managed centers: The importance of cost analysis. *Outcomes Management for Nursing Practice, 4*(3), 124–128.

Vonderheid, S., Pohl, J. M., Barkauskas, V. H., Hughes-Cromwick, P., & Gift, D. (March, 2002). *Performance of academic nurse-managed primary care centers.* Paper presented at the 26th Annual Research Conference of the Midwest Nursing Research Society, Chicago.

Walker, P. H. (1995). Faculty practice: Interest, issues and impact. In J. Fitzpatrick & J. Stevenson (Eds.), *Annual Review of Nursing Research* (pp. 217–235). New York: Springer.

Watson, L. J. (1996). A national profile of nursing centers: Arenas for advanced practice. *Nurse Practitioner, 21*(3), 72–73, 79 ff.

Zuckerman, H. S., Kaluzny, A. D., & Ricketts, T. C. (1995). Strategic alliances: A worldwide phenomenon comes to health care. In A. D. Kaluzny, H. S. Zuckerman, T. C. Ricketts, & G. B. Walton (Eds.), *Partners for the dance: Forming strategic alliances in health care* (pp. 1–18). Ann Arbor, MI: Health Administration Press.

Chapter 13

Building a Critical Mass:
The Penn Macy Initiative

Norma M. Lang, Lois K. Evans,
Beth Ann Swan, and
Rebecca A. Snyder Phillips

Schools of nursing are expected to provide the thought leadership for solving pressing problems in delivering health care, evolving nursing science, and preparing the next generations of practitioners and leaders. The growing gap between academic and clinical arenas in nursing has impeded the development and implementation of new knowledge in the discipline. The deliberate integration of research, education, and clinical care to meet multiple goals, especially by schools of nursing in research intensive environments, has great promise for closing this gap. The widespread adoption of this new integration, however, is hampered by schools' deficiencies in capacity, common focus and direction, visibility and voice, and critical mass. This chapter describes a major national initiative designed to address these deficits and to help propel the building of a critical mass of 21 schools of nursing in research intensive environments engaged in academic nursing practice. Detailed description of the Penn Macy Initiative to Advance Academic Nursing Practice (PMIAANP) may be found in two publications (Lang, Evans, & Swan, 2002; Evans, Swan, & Lang, 2003). A summary of structure, components, and outcomes, including key readiness indicators for launching academic nursing practice agendas, are included here.

COMPONENTS OF THE PENN MACY INITIATIVE

Background

The Josiah Macy, Jr, Foundation of New York went into partnership with the University of Pennsylvania School of Nursing (UPSON) to mount the PMIAANP that was aimed at growing the science of nursing by integrating the tripartite mission in academic practice and fostering replication of successful academic practices in schools of nursing nationally. A 3-year grant of $500,000 from the Macy Foundation provided for a planning year and 2 years of implementation and evaluation. UPSON's own struggles, experiences, and successes in expanding an academic nursing practice agenda to include a network of school-owned and operated practices provided the impetus for the initiative (Evans, Jenkins, & Buhler-Wilkerson, 2003; see also Chapters 4 & 5). Recognizing the lengthy time it takes for research to be integrated into practice (Lang, 2001; Eisenberg, 2001), and wishing to help jump start this process to improve the quality and effectiveness of health care, UPSON envisioned that a critical mass of schools in research-intensive environments with their strong programs of research, advanced practice education, and leadership would have the best chances for success. Since schools of nursing would require assistance with capacity building in order to sustain their academic nursing practice initiatives, the PMIAANP was designed to provide opportunities for participating schools from across the country to learn from one another on site and to receive support over a subsequent one year period in achieving their individualized goals.

Structure

The PMIAANP was established in 1998 to help schools of nursing develop and advance academic practice. The planning year was used to sharpen the focus; identify the target schools; design the application, content, materials, consultation and evaluation plan; and recruit the first of two groups of participant schools. Aiming to create a critical mass of schools in research-intensive environments engaged in academic nursing practice expansion, an overall goal of reaching at least 20 of the (then) approximately 100 schools in Carnegie I or II universities was set. Five major components were used to help facilitate participant schools' development: self-assessment and application, an intensive summer institute, a 12-month period of individualized consultation and networking, the Senior Fellows Exchange, and self-evaluation. Each of these will be briefly described.

Self-Assessment and Application. To obtain the 20% critical-mass target—ten participant schools each year—deans of schools in research intensive settings and/or having a doctoral program in nursing, and/or top ranking in National Institutes of Health (NIH) research grants were apprised of the opportunity to apply. The application itself required a detailed self-assessment by applicant schools as to their level of academic practice development to date, goals for further expansion, and their related strengths and challenges. The data included interest in and history with academic practice development; relationship of academic nursing practice to mission, vision, and strategic plans; placement of academic practice in the table of organization; relevant APT policies; research and program funding experience in academic practice; expertise in business, finance and reimbursement for practice; analysis of strengths and potential barriers for achieving goals; description of current practices; and specific objectives for participating in the PMI. While the review process attempted to select schools with similar levels of readiness in order to facilitate learning, it was recognized at the outset that each applicant school was unique in its set of attributes and strengths. Table 13.1 lists the participant schools for each year.

TABLE 13.1   Schools Participating in the Penn Macy Initiative (N = 21)

1999	2000
New York University	Pennsylvania State University
Temple University	Rutgers University
University of California at Los Angeles	University of Florida
University of Colorado	University of Iowa
University of Kentucky	University of Michigan
University of Rochester	University of Minnesota
University of Texas	University of Nebraska
University of Virginia	Vanderbilt University
University of Washington	Virginia Commonwealth University
University of Wisconsin-Madison	Wayne State University
	West Virginia University

Five Day Intensive Summer Institute. Participant schools were asked to name an Academic Practice Resource Team (APRT) composed of up to three persons representing the perspectives of nursing faculty in research and practice, health care business management or equivalent, and academic financial administration. Learning with an aim of creating change in an organization requires more than one "champion," as has been shown in previous initiatives (Phillips, 1997; Inouye, Acampora, Miller, Fulmer, Hurst, & Cooney, 1993). Further, at least these three perspectives were deemed essential for moving forward an academic practice agenda. With 10–11 schools participating in each year's Institute, a maximum of 25–30 participants was believed ideal for the tailored participative model, based on the experience of the Johnson and Johnson–Wharton Fellows Program in Management for Nurse Executives (Rovin & Ginsburg, 1988) after which the Institute was modeled.

The Summer Institute addressed content areas believed to be critical to successful academic nursing practice expansion. While specific content differed each year, dependent on the expressed needs and goals of participants, several general categories were included. These were focused on the intricate and tenuous relationship of academic practice and research, academic practice outcomes and models, organizational infrastructure and resources for supporting academic practice, and vision for the future. Content leaders were primarily professors, clinical faculty/leaders, administrators, and board members from UPSON/UP. In year two, selected senior fellows from the first year of the PMIAANP also participated. A combination of lecture-discussion, audiovisuals, small group discussions, and field visits were used.

Individualized Consultation and Networking. Having refined their own 1-year goals for academic practice expansion during course of the Institute, the teams could each request from the Penn Macy Faculty up to 5 hours of individualized consultation related to reaching their goals over the next year. The schools' goals included attaining fiscal viability; building infrastructure; structuring organization for practice; integrating research and education with practice; and providing for APT criteria in support of scholarly practice endeavors. Peer networking, begun after the forming of the Institute, was enhanced through a Web site that hosted chat rooms, discussion boards, and knowledge center; a listserv; and follow up meetings (Lang, Evans, & Swan, 2002). As described elsewhere (Evans, Swan, & Lang, 2003), two thirds of the schools used an average of 3 hours each for consultation in such areas as finance, organization, research, and clinical issues. In comparison to the electronic methods, personal networking was used more extensively and effectively by the senior fellows.

Senior Fellows Exchange. At the end of the Summer Institute, each team member was awarded a certificate and named Penn Macy Fellow in Academic Nursing Practice. Many were able to meet informally midyear during the American Association of Colleges of Nursing (AACN) Faculty Practice Conference. Fellows were invited formally to return at the end of the year to share lessons learned with peer Fellows. The topics clustered around common themes: models for academic nursing practice, integrating research and practice, database development, financial survival, and faculty incentives. Three of the 21 schools chose not to participate in the exchange because of issues related to changes in their missions and/or operations.

Self-Evaluation. APRTs were asked to evaluate each component of the 5-day Summer Institute on a daily basis and at the conclusion of the 5 days. This feedback was used to make midcourse corrections in methodology and content as well as to shape the Institute for the following year. Further, in addition to the schools' self-assessment that formed the application process, each team was asked to firm up their 1-year goals for academic practice during the 5 days at the Institute, and then they were to track their progress toward goal achievement through quarterly and 1-year reports. In addition, schools were asked to track achievement in each of 5 areas deemed critical to academic practice development—namely, fiscal viability, planning and operations, educational integration, research integration, and organizational viability.

EXPERIENCE AND OUTCOMES

Participants

The 21 participating schools represented a range of expertise and experience with an organizational commitment to academic nursing practice (Evans, Swan, & Lang, 2002). The majority (86%) were in public universities. Participant schools reported a broad spectrum of practice history, some dating from the 1970s; others were more recent. The average was 13 years, and the period tended to be longer for schools with long-established graduate programs. For just over three quarters, practice was a component of their written mission statement, 90% addressed practice in faculty APT criteria, and for 86%, practice had a place on the organization chart. They described having a range of practice models: a mixed portfolio that included contract/joint appointment and/or partnerships and/or full financial risk practices was reported by 76%, and 81% reported owning risk practices.

These experiences also represented a mix of experience with managed care, fee for service, and contractual means of support. Most schools had been successful in securing grant support for practice or related educational programs, but fewer reported funded research related to their academic practices. Regarding the composition of the APRTs, most demonstrated some mix in perspectives and were also varied in faculty level and rank, faculty responsibilities, and levels and types of administrative personnel. Nearly half of the deans also attended at least a portion of the 5-day Summer Institute.

Evaluation

The evaluation process and findings are described in detail elsewhere (Evans, Swan, & Lang, 2003). Participants generally gave high marks to the Institute and its content and speakers, as well as to other components of the PMIAANP. In particular, they found the peer networking to be especially useful.

The quarterly and annual self reports were viewed as meeting two major needs. In addition to helping evaluate the outcomes of the PMIAANP, the process of completing the evaluation in itself provided important data to participating schools that they could use for decision making, strategic planning, midcourse corrections, and so on. While annual reports were received from all 21 schools, quarterly progress reports were received only from some, and, like the quality of the applications themselves, these reports differed in level of detail and specificity.

In general, each school made progress in reaching their goals and in achieving change in critical indicators. School achievement in each of the five critical indicators (practice fiscal viability, planning and operations, education integration, research integration, and organizational viability) and individualized goals were categorized as being at, above or below expected levels. Overall, best progress was attained in the two areas of planning/operations and organizational viability, while minimal progress was reported in research integration.

Accomplishments

Accomplishments were summarized for each of the five critical indicator areas. Examples included diversification of practice portfolios (fiscal viability); implementation of clinical information systems and tracking quality indicators and fiscal benchmarks (planning and operations); implementation of new practice-derived courses (educational integration); integration of funded research projects into existing practice settings (research integration); and organization of faculty practice plans and revision of APT criteria (organizational viability).

KEY INDICATORS OF SUCCESS

Given the differences in schools at the onset and also the variability in their movement during the year, a closer look at those with the higher and lower levels of progression was undertaken (See Evans, Swan, & Lang, 2003). Seven of the 16 characteristics thought to be important to successful development in academic practice expansion were demonstrated by all schools that progressed beyond expectations. In contrast, no characteristics were demonstrated by every school at the minimal progress level. It is believed that structural characteristics—practice in the mission statement and long range strategic plan, history of faculty practice, and APT criteria that address practice—are important but not essential, in and of themselves, to assure successful expansion of the academic nursing practice agenda. Likewise displaying an overall readiness to mount a new venture—clear goals, tight application, achievable strategies—is insufficient alone.

Three major points were concluded:

1. While key characteristics are important, it is the unique mix of characteristics—in the context of the schools' individual history, location in a particular institution and healthcare environment, commitment and vision of the dean and other leaders, composition and mission of the faculty, school's strategic plans, and access to external and internal resources at a point in time—that is critical to success.
2. The degree of understanding a school has of its unique context, then, is essential to readiness and ability to take advantage of opportunities.
3. Of all the areas involved in academic nursing practice expansion— financial stability notwithstanding—it is the integration of research and practice that appears to remain most challenging.

CHALLENGES FOR THE FUTURE

Over a 2-year period, PMIAANP prepared a critical mass of fellows in academic nursing practice from 21 research-intensive schools of nursing across the United States. The fellows, themselves, have been increasingly visible at the faculty practice conferences of the AACN and other organizations, have provided consultation to peer schools, and have published results of their own journeys on the academic nursing practice path. Following the first 2 Summer Institutes, UPSON continued to hold an annual 2-day conference called Academic Nursing Practice—Creating the Evidence Base; maintained an electronic listserv, Web-based knowledge center and Web site, and provided fee-for-service consultation in areas related to academic practice. Leadership emerging from among the fellows for moving the academic nursing practice agenda forward gives hope for the continued future of this work and provides evidence for the important role of PMI in providing impetus, leadership, and resources for academic nursing practice in the years to come.

REFERENCES

Eisenberg, J. M. (2001). Putting research to work and enhancing the impact of health services research. *Health Services Research, 36*(2), x–xvii.

Evans, L. K., Jenkins, M., & Buhler-Wilkerson, K. (2003). Academic nursing practice: Implications for policy. In M. D. Mezey, D. O. McGivern, & E. Sullivan-Marx (Eds.), *Nurse practitioners: Evolution of advanced practice* (4th ed., pp. 443–470). New York: Springer.

Evans, L. K., Swan, B. A., & Lang, N. M. (2003). Evaluation of the Penn Macy Initiative to advance academic nursing practice. *Journal of Professional Nursing, 19*(1), 8–16.

Inouye, S. K., Acampora, D., Miller, R. L., Fulmer, T., Hurst, L. D., et al. (1993). The Yale Geriatric Care Program: A model of care to prevent functional decline in hospitalized elderly patients. *Journal of American Geriatrics Society, 41,* 1345–1352.

Lang, N. M. (2001). Developing knowledge for policy and practice for the 21st century. *Nursing Leadership Forum, 5,* 74–81.

Lang, N. M., Evans, L. K., & Swan, B. A. (2002). Penn Macy Initiative to Advance Academic Nursing Practice. *Journal of Professional Nursing, 18*(2), 63–69.

Phillips, R. S. (1997). Distance learning initiative 'cuts the edge' on providing continuing education to nursing home professionals in remote and distant areas of Pennsylvania. *University of Pennsylvania Institute on Aging Newsletter, 6*(3), 1, 7.

Rovin, S., & Ginsberg, L. T. (1988). Johnson & Johnson–Wharton Fellows Program in Management for Nurses. *Nursing Economic$, 6*(2), 78–82.

Looking Ahead . . .

" The decade of the 1990s was a time for dreaming, and for strategizing ways to realize those dreams . . . " Thus began the first chapter of this book. Much occurred over that decade that was both hopeful and disappointing for academic nursing practice. Yet those events, some of which have been described in the preceding chapters, form the experience base out of which the future will unfold.

Health care planning has oscillated between bold visions that seem impossible to implement and incremental actions that absorb and overwhelm. We need to better link 'dreaming' and 'strategic acting.' When Steven Ross, the creator of Time Warner, was a teenager, he received the following deathbed advice from his father (Creator of Time Warner, 1992): "There are those who work all day, and there are those who dream all day, and those who spend an hour daydreaming before setting to work to fulfill these dreams. Go into the third category because there is virtually no competition" (p. 12). We invite readers to join together in that third category to explore the kind of movement nursing needs to lead and be a part of to make the ideas so richly laid out by our colleagues come together in a sustainable, valuable way. Draw on the preceding chapters, assemble interested colleagues both within and outside of nursing, and discover what you can do locally and nationally. What will emerge over the decades to come remains to be seen as evidence accumulates of the influence of academic nursing practice on health care and on the profession.

T. S. Eliot (1971) once wrote, "What we call the beginning is often the end. And to make an end is to make a beginning. The end is where we start from" (p. 144). The next phase of our future has already begun . . .

Lois and Norma

REFERENCES

Creator of Time Warner, Steven J. Ross, is Dead at 65 (12 December, 1992). *New York Times*, p. 12.

Eliot, T. S. (1971). Four Quartets: Little Gidding. *The complete poems and plays 1909–1950*. New York: Harcourt, Brace and World, Inc.

Index

Springer Publishing Company

From the Springer Series: Teaching of Nursing…

Community-Based Nursing Education

The Experiences of Eight Schools of Nursing

Peggy S. Matteson, RNC, PhD, Editor

"Just as each neighborhood is unique so must be every community-based nursing education program. Each of the programs (described in this book) demonstrates a unique way in which the principles of community based education …may be implemented either in a portion of, or across the curriculum. The book is a testimony to creative and innovative projects that emerge when creative faculty and community partners work together."

—from the **Preface**

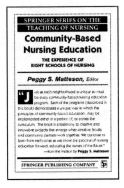

Contents:

2000   256pp   0-8261-1323-0   hardcover

536 Broadway, New York, NY 10012
Order Toll-Free: 877-687-7476 • Order On-line: www.springerpub.com

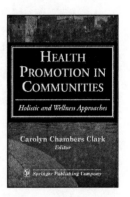

Springer Publishing Company

Clinical Excellence for Nurse Practitioners
The International Journal of NPACE

Joellen W. Hawkins, RNC, PhD, FAAN, Editor
Susan Daggett Bennett, MSN, RN, CS-ANP
Frances Medaglia Dwyer, PhD, RN, CS-GNP
Richard S. Ferri, PhD, ANP, ACRN, FAAN
Joyce Pulcini, PhD, RN, CS-PNP, Associate Editors

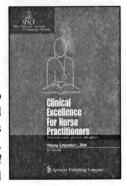

This quarterly is a peer-reviewed journal designed to facilitate communication about practice, education, and research for advanced practice nurses. Each issue presents columns on clinical practice, clinical studies, pharmacology, policy and regulatory issues, and APN education. *Clinical Excellence for Nurse Practitioners* is the official publication of NPACE (Nurse Practitioner Associates for Continuing Education).

Sample Contents:
Editorial
- Musings on Attitudes and Their Effects on Our Health and Well-Being: You're Only as Old as You Feel or Behave, *Joellen W. Hawkins*

Clinical Practice
- Diagnosis and Treatment of Persons With Restless Legs Syndrome, *Norma G. Cuellar*
- Breast Cancer Screening Behavior Among Low-Income and Minority Women, *Mary Kerans*

Clinical Studies
- Experiences of Adoptive Parents of Children With Fetal Alcohol Syndrome, *Joan Granitsas*
- The Incubator Model: Is It Effective Prenatal Care, *Brandy L. Worley, Linda F. C. Bullock, and Elizabeth Geden*
- The Availability and Accessibility of Gynecological and Reproductive Services for Women With Developmental Disabilities: A Nursing Perspective, *Catharine Kopac, and Joni Fritz*

ISSN 1085-2360 • Volume 8, 2004 • Published 4 times per year

536 Broadway, New York, NY 10012
Order Toll-Free: 877-687-7476 • Order On-line: www.springerpub.com

Springer Publishing Company

Annual Review of Nursing Education

Marilyn H. Oermann, PhD, RN, FAAN, Editor
Kathleen T. Heinrich, PhD, RN, Associate Editor

Interested in the latest trends in nursing education written by the nurse educators pioneering these innovations? Then welcome to the **Annual Review of Nursing Education.** This **Review** describes educational strategies you can adapt to your own settings and is written for educators in associate, baccalaureate, and graduate nursing programs, staff development, and continuing education. The goal of the **Review** is to keep educators updated on recent innovations in nursing education across all settings.

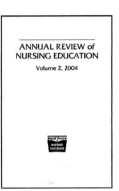

ANNUAL REVIEW of
NURSING EDUCATION
Volume 2, 2004

Partial Contents Volume 2:

2004   400pp   0-8261-2445-3   hardcover

536 Broadway, New York, NY 10012
Order Toll-Free: 877-687-7476 • Order On-line: www.springerpub.com

3